Praise for Harriet Washington's

INFECTIOUS MADNESS

"An enthusiastic report on research suggesting that some mental illnesses are partly caused by pathogens."

— *New York Times Book Review* Editors' Choice

"It used to be obvious what caused mental illness—depravity, a rotten soul, being in cahoots with the Devil. Or maybe just terrible mothering. We've escaped this primordial muck of attribution, learning that mental illnesses are biological disorders, complete with chemical and structural abnormalities in the brain, and with risk factors ranging from genes, hormones, and fetal life to socioeconomic status. This superb book reviews the novel realization that infectious pathogens, and the immune system's response to them, can be risk factors for mental illness as well. The book has a broad, exciting range, considering 'contagion' in both the reductive sense as well as in the expansive societal manner. This is fascinating material and Harriet Washington is a great writer—clear and accessible, witty, probing, and able to dissect the controversies in this field with great objectivity."

— Robert Sapolsky, author of *Why Zebras Don't Get Ulcers*

"Intriguing.... Very well-written." — Dr. Mehmet Oz

"In making the infectious pitch, Washington rightly argues that it strengthens the case for abandoning the Cartesian dualism that separates mind from body and leads to stigma and fear. It's acceptable to study how infection and immunity affect the brain, but only as part of a larger agenda to understand the brain in all its plasticity and complexity. Conclusion: an unproven but undoubtedly provocative case. Expect dissent and discussion." — *Kirkus Reviews*

"A fascinating exploration of how common infections can affect mental illness."   —Shanda Deziel, *Chatelaine*

"Your views on the causes of mental illness will be forever altered when you read this profoundly humane and transformative book."
—Carl Hart, PhD, associate professor of psychology, Columbia University

"You'll never look at your household pet the same way again."
—*New York Post*

"A thought-provoking book....Washington convincingly argues that infections cause 10 to 15 percent of mental disease."
—Karen Springen, *Booklist*

"*Infectious Madness* is a fascinating book about the role of infectious diseases in mental illness. Washington challenges us to expand our view of the causes, prevention, and treatment of emotional disorders. I highly recommend it!"
—Alvin F. Poussaint, MD, professor of psychiatry, Harvard Medical School

"Terrifying and comforting in equal measure. *Infectious Madness* will inspire healthy debate and, Washington hopes, bold new strategies for prevention and treatment."   —Priscilla Gilman, *More*

"An impressive array of technical research is presented in a readable style....Recommended for fans of science journalism and readers interested in the next 'hot topic' in biological psychiatry."
—Antoinette Brinkman, *Library Journal*

"With *Infectious Madness,* Harriet Washington sounds a much-needed alarm—although not a welcome one. Turning old-fashioned germ theory inside out, she explains that we humans are the slow-moving interlopers in a world of microbes. And it's not just our health but our instincts, desires, feelings, and even our grasp on reality that are at stake."

—Philip Alcabes, professor of public health, Adelphi University, author of *Dread: How Fear and Fantasy Have Fueled Epidemics from the Black Death to Avian Flu*

"In *Infectious Madness,* Harriet Washington confirms her position as one of our most thought-provoking medical writers. Led by Washington on a whirlwind tour of early modern medicine in the eighteenth century, germ theory, Western anorexia, African sleeping sickness, schizophrenia, and everywhere else, we will forever be unable to think of our microbial environment in the same way. The same, for that matter, might be said of our view of the social environment in which the collective enterprise of medicine transpires."

—Samuel Roberts, PhD, director, Columbia University Institute for Research in African-American Studies, and associate professor of sociomedical sciences, Columbia University Mailman School of Public Health

INFECTIOUS MADNESS

INFECTIOUS MADNESS

THE SURPRISING SCIENCE OF
HOW WE "CATCH" MENTAL ILLNESS

HARRIET A. WASHINGTON

Little, Brown Spark
New York Boston London

Little, Brown Spark / Little, Brown and Company
Hachette Book Group
1290 Avenue of the Americas, New York, NY 10104
littlebrownspark.com

Originally published in hardcover by Little, Brown and Company, October 2015
First paperback edition, October 2016

Little, Brown Spark is an imprint of Little, Brown and Company, a division of Hachette Book Group, Inc. The Little, Brown Spark name and logo are trademarks of Hachette Book Group, Inc.

The publisher is not responsible for websites (or their content) that are not owned by the publisher.

The Hachette Speakers Bureau provides a wide range of authors for speaking events. To find out more, go to hachettespeakersbureau.com or call (866) 376-6591.

Photograph on page 46 courtesy of Frey at last; page 48, courtesy of Government of South Australia; page 181, courtesy of Randall Bytwerk; page 202, by Greg and Mary Beth Dimijian.

ISBN 978-0-316-27780-8 (hc) / 978-0-316-27781-5 (pb)
Library of Congress Control Number 2015935999

10 9 8 7 6 5 4 3

LSC-C

Printed in the United States of America

For Pete

The highest activities of consciousness have their origins in physical occurrences of the brain just as the loveliest melodies are not too sublime to be expressed by notes.

— W. SOMERSET MAUGHAM

Contents

Introduction   3

Chapter 1: Germ Theory Redux: The Acquisition
               of Mental Illness   9

Chapter 2: The Fetus as Battleground:
               Early Exposure and Psychiatric Fate   38

Chapter 3: Growing Pains: "Catching" Anorexia,
               Obsessive-Compulsive Disorder,
               and Tourette's   76

Chapter 4: Gut Feelings: The Brain in Your Belly   125

Chapter 5: Microbial Culture: Pathogens and the
               Shaping of Societies   158

Chapter 6: Winning at Evolutionary Chess:
               Strategies to Outwit Pathogens   192

Chapter 7: Tropical Madness: Infection and
               Neglect in the Developing World   225

Afterword   251

Acknowledgments   257

Notes   261

Index   289

INFECTIOUS
MADNESS

Introduction

Gazing into the night sky with its seemingly numberless stars evokes our sense of infinity, but if you seek the ultimate multitude, look closer to home. What lies at our feet and within us dwarfs the heavenly spectacle, yet we need our imaginations— or a powerful microscope—to see it: microscopic bugs, not stars, dominate the galaxies. The earth alone holds five million times more microbes than there are suns in the universe. It is home to five *nonillion* infinitesimal beings—that's a 5 followed by 30 zeros.

Five million bacteria teem in every teaspoonful of seawater, accompanied by fifty million viruses. This makes viruses the most common life form in the seas, and no wonder: viruses infect most other living organisms, including bacteria.

Microbes do more than infect us, however; they *are* us, in the sense that we harbor more microbes than human cells. Your intestines alone provide a home for one hundred *trillion* viruses, fungi, protozoans, and—mostly—bacteria. These single-celled guests outnumber your cells ten to one.

Microbes thickly coat our skin, eyes, and genitals and cover the surfaces of our mouths; they specialize in specific areas of the body. Staphylococci colonize the skin, and lactobacilli coat the vagina. And that's just on the surface; ten thousand different species of organisms thickly populate your gut. Just as our genes make up our genomes, these microbial fellow travelers make up our microbiomes, which constantly adjust in type and numbers on different sites on the body and different sites on the globe.

And our health, including our mental health, changes with them.

Your microbiome has an astonishing power to keep you healthy—or ill. From the beginning, internal microbes guide your immune system's development. Your gut also possesses its own "brain." It houses a network, dubbed the *enteric nervous system,* or *ENS,* that contains a thousand times more neurons than your brain does. Its weight is twice that of your brain and it sends neurotransmitters that help direct your brain's activities.

During birth we acquire microbes from our mothers that confer immunity and may dictate our future health, from struggles with weight to a propensity to schizophrenia. As we grow, we acquire more pathogens and beneficial microbial "friends" that tip our odds of developing or avoiding everything from ulcers to heart disease to cervical cancer to obsessive-compulsive disorder.

The relationship between disease and microbes was first proposed in the seventeenth century, but the evidence and basic standards for the proof of infectious-disease causation weren't laid down until 1883, when the German bacteriologists Robert Koch and Friedrich Loeffler provided the first evidence that tiny, invisible microbes enter the body and cause diseases; this is *germ theory.*

The microscope enabled scientists to see the pathogens, document them, and, in doing so, disprove popular beliefs, such as that sinful behavior invites illness or that poisonous vapors called *miasmas* cause disease.

The uncontrollable dancing movements of St. Anthony's fire, once ascribed to satanic influence, are now known to result from *Claviceps purpurea,* a fungus that infects rye. Malaria is now known to be caused not by bad air but by a single-celled plasmodium, a parasite of the female *Anopheles* mosquito.

Contemporary researchers on five continents continue to

unmask microbial roots of illness, and they now recognize that events as seemingly trivial as a sore throat or a case of measles — or even the flu — can breed anorexia, Tourette's, obsessive-compulsive disorder, or schizophrenia. Researchers in the field estimate that infectious organisms cause from 10 percent to 75 percent of some serious mental disorders.

In 1997, I glimpsed the extent to which mental illnesses are connected to infection when I happened upon an Italian medical-journal article that linked schizophrenia to bornavirus, which causes a fatal encephalitis in Central European sheep and horses. It asked whether humans acquire the virus from horses and whether such infections can cause schizophrenia. The article found a strong correlation between infection and illness, but no proof. Thus, it was inconclusive, and so were subsequent studies, as I learned when I called the investigators.

I was disappointed, but my curiosity was piqued as I searched for evidence of causal connections between infection and mental illness. I quickly found them, but many were lodged in the past. General paresis, cases of which once filled one of every five New York City asylum beds, is caused by a familiar disease: syphilis. When scientists discovered that penicillin cured syphilis, they also discovered a cure for this common mental disease. Now one must travel to the developing world to see a case.

In 1997, I learned of Paul Ewald, a visionary evolutionary biologist whose work describes a second wave of germ theory. He has elegantly argued for the unperceived importance of infection as an explanation of much human disease. Bacteria, viruses, fungi, and other infectious agents are responsible for many of the illnesses that we have long ascribed to genetics, behaviors, and even personality types. Cervical cancer, for example, was long chalked up to sexual immoderation but is now known to be triggered by certain strains of the human papillomavirus, just as the hepatitis C virus causes hepatitis C. Ninety percent of ulcers, which were long attributed to unmanaged stress and treated with milk, antacids, and the acid-lowering drug Tagamet, are actually caused by a bacterium, *Helicobacter pylori*, although stress may impair an ulcer's healing. Many heart attacks, long ascribed to aggressive, hostile, type A personalities, are now recognized as the legacy of the bacterium *Chlamydophila pneumoniae* as well as various gut bacteria.

In 1997 I also discovered the work of Dr. Susan Swedo, who proposed an intriguing syndrome fingering Group A streptococcal bacteria, or GAS bacteria, as the culprit in children who developed symptoms of anorexia, obsessive-compulsive disorder, or Tourette's in the wake of strep throats. She was actively seeking proof and a mechanism in human studies with scores of adolescents, many of whom had been brought to her clinics at the National Institute of Mental Health by their worried parents. I reported on these exciting developments in *Psychology Today*, but aside from Swedo's fledgling human studies, I found little contemporary evidence, just tantalizing correlations between infections and madness.

I periodically looked into the state of research linking microbes and mental disorders, and in 2013, I realized that it was burgeoning. With the acknowledgment of epigenetics, scientists moved away from exclusively genetic models of disease, including mental disease, and this made it easier to contemplate microbial causes and risk factors.

The pioneering research of scientists like Michael Gershon and Martin J. Blaser laid the groundwork for an emphasis on gut microbes that resulted in 2008's Human Microbiome Project, a $115 million enterprise that sought to discern the microbial causes of health and illnesses, including depression, autism, and obesity.

Since the early 1970s, when Freud's theories of mental illness were ascendant, prescient scientists like E. Fuller Torrey, director of the Stanley Medical Research Institute, and Robert Yolken, of Johns Hopkins, had rejected the belief that schizophrenia and other psychoses were exclusively the result of social and psychological dynamics. Instead, they had looked for answers in biology, specifically in microbial assaults on the immune and nervous systems. By 2013, mental-illness researchers had largely abandoned Freud to join the duo in exploring neurophysiology.

As a result of this sea change in research directions, we are approaching critical mass: a paradigm shift that replaces psychosocial factors with biological ones as the cause of mental illness. Most (not all) involved researchers think that microbes constitute just one risk factor; genetics, stress, psychological factors, and social dynamics are still important. In fact, most experts who hazard an informed guess about their relative importance suggest that infections cause 10 to 15 percent of mental disease. That may sound like a small number at first, but it is quite significant, especially when we consider, within that statistic, the many lives lost through suicide or early death and the even greater number of lives lost to profound disability.

Moreover, Yolken reminds us that immense numbers of mentally ill in poor and developing nations go undiagnosed, and we are not even aware of a greater number of microbes that undoubtedly exist in such areas; it is a mathematical certainty that some of them pose mental-health threats.

This book traces the growing evidence of microbial triggers of mental disease in infants, adolescents, adults, and people in the developing world. In describing the infinite variety of pathogenic mental disorders, it also interrogates the nature of proof, as opposed to mere correlation, and proposes that traditional mechanisms for establishing proof must be supplemented by modern tools and strategies. It examines the equally outmoded and simplistic notion of the "war" between man and his microbial hangers-on and suggests that our seek-and-destroy approach to pathogen control must be replaced by more nuanced strategies; we are involved in a chess game, not a brute battle to the death.

This book urges readers to employ the reasoning scientists have applied to physical illness to microbial mental illness. I'll show through historical examples that we have been loath to follow the facts that establish microbial causes and that our biases and antiquated habits of thought have resulted in our clinging to scientifically untenable and ineffective theories and treatments that have cost many their sanity and their lives.

Not only do microbes play a surprising role in our tastes and preferences—some acquired tastes seem related to our microbial exposure, as I'll explore—they also shape our societies. *Infectious Madness* discusses research demonstrating how microbes influence our collective behavior, shedding light on issues that go far beyond individual mental health. It looks at how the poor and medically underserved suffer far worse mental health than the rest of the population, in part because neither their pathogens nor their mental ailments receive appropriate scientific treatment. As it turns out, microbes shed light on some of the most mysterious and vital questions we face: Why are some societies more xenophobic than others? Why do some peoples tolerate or even encourage stranger violence, such as lynching, the Holocaust, or ethnic genocide in Bosnia and Rwanda?

In short, *Infectious Madness* endeavors to relate through the prescient work of visionary scientists how microbes rule not only the world, but also our minds.

CHAPTER 1

Germ Theory Redux: The Acquisition of Mental Illness

A new scientific truth does not triumph by convincing its opponents and making them see the light, but rather because its opponents eventually die, and a new generation grows up that is familiar with it.

— MAX PLANCK

"When I was a student in the 1960s, I once saw a man in the final stage of syphilis," recalls English writer John Cornwell. "He was a patient on a psychiatric ward in London where I was working. White-haired, olive-skinned, emaciated, without a name or known country of origin, he had been picked up from a gutter in the London docks."

The man lived in a state hospital for the mentally ill, where he was cared for by a kind but resigned staff. "He stood all day in the corridor leaning against the wall, doing a slow-motion foot shuffle." The man, Cornwell tells us, was more than psychologically impaired. He could not hear or speak and seemed oblivious to his surroundings. "The ward charge nurse assured me that he was 'unlucky, the last of his kind.' He had not been given treatment in time to halt the final devastation of the disease."[1]

Cornwell's account reminded me of a patient I had encountered while working in an upstate New York county hospital in the 1960s. He was probably in his early sixties, but he looked younger, thanks to his vacant gaze and unfurrowed brow. Dressed in khaki pants and a T-shirt,[2] he was gently propped in front of a peeling greenish wall every day, and he remained there, a slight smile playing about his lips, his equanimity undisturbed by the chaos and noise of the behavioral renegades with whom he shared the dayroom. Once, he was placed too close to the naked bulb of a torchère lamp whose shade had been lost in some forgotten drama, but when a staff member moved it to a safe distance, he neither averted his eyes nor tracked the aggressive glare. He was blind. He was also deaf, unable to speak or communicate, and he showed no signs of being able to reason or remember. He was reduced to someone who ate and defecated, who was bathed and dressed and shuffled along to nowhere with utter indifference. No one ever visited him.

What had happened to this man? The aide shepherding him to dinner whispered, "He's got paresis, and it has destroyed his brain. It's an old disease, you never see it now. He was treated with penicillin, but they can't bring back the lost function."

Lost. I hung on the adjective, which seemed to capture his condition so perfectly. Then I did a double take. "Penicillin? An antibiotic? For a severe mental disorder?" The aide shrugged as she and her charge moved on.

The antibiotic was in order because general paresis, a form of neurosyphilis, is seen in the late stages of syphilis and can emerge twenty to thirty years after the initial infection. Because it attacks in a very nonspecific manner, the neurosyphilis infection can appear in many different ways and damage many different areas of the brain. Whatever region comes under fire by the bacteria and their antibodies determines the disease's signs and symptoms, which are legion. In both Cornwell's patient and in the upstate New York man I observed, aural and visual systems had been destroyed and motor functions reduced to stereotyped residual movements. This damage can cause delusions, hallucinations, a diminished ability to think or speak, personality changes, impaired judgment, anger, irritability, and a sad or depressed mood. Both short-term and long-term memory may eventually disappear. There are physical consequences too, including changes in the pupil of the eye, overactive reflexes, sharp pains, a slow degeneration of the neurons' ability to transmit messages (somewhat like that seen in multiple sclerosis), and profound muscle weakness, all of which eventually relegate paresis sufferers to bed.

The New York man was treated in a general hospital, but the man with paresis whom Cornwell encountered in England was being treated by psychiatrists in a mental institution, as befitted his profound dementia and psychological and mental losses.[3] If one had to choose between the two labels, this clearly was mental illness. Or was it? Given that a paresis patient is dogged by the loss of control over his movements, loss of vision, and other physical problems, and given that all this carnage resulted from a bacterial infection, was this not a physical disorder? For that matter, does one have to choose?

"There may be said to be two classes of people in the world," mused Algonquin Round Table habitué Robert Benchley in 1920, "those who constantly divide the people of the world into two classes, and those who do not."[4] Physicians belong to the first group. They embrace the long-standing mind-body dualism that insists that mental disorders solely affect the mind, and physical disorders are the product of distorted physiology.

The fact that psychiatric diseases are now routinely located in brain dysfunction doesn't resolve the issue, because this acknowledgment doesn't necessarily represent a dissolution of the imaginary boundary between the physical and the mental. Instead, this stance often entails a belief in two distinct species of "mind." In one, consciousness and mental disorders are created by and dependent on the functioning of the brain, a sort of ghostly extension of the brain into psychic space. The other mind is viewed as completely separate from the brain. But without a specific indication of precisely which mind is meant, the scientific literature is often maddeningly fuzzy and unhelpful.

To what extent is automatically ascribing mental disease to psychological trauma and genetic determinism and physical disease to tangible environmental causes just a lazy habit of thought?

For ancient Greeks, the distinction between psychological and medical illness was not the most salient or definitive characteristic of disorders. In Hippocrates's disease taxonomy, mania, melancholia, and hysteria were treated with the same humoral-imbalance corrections that he prescribed for physical illnesses.

At the other extreme, there's a long history of attributing psychosis to moral failure. In Deuteronomy 28:27–29, rebellious Israelites were threatened with insanity. "The Lord will smite you with madness, blindness and with bewilderment of heart," it promises. Medieval scholars and theologians believed madness was spiritually induced, either by a failure of faith or by a punishment from the gods, a theory that died hard and that, arguably, persists in pockets of fundamentalism and faith healers.

However, by the time of the Renaissance, physicians and other Western medical experts placed mental diseases firmly in the fold of physical ailments and treated them as such.[5] This view persisted for centuries. "From the Renaissance until the second half of the 18th century," wrote R. E. Kendell in the *British Journal of Psychiatry*, "melancholia and other forms of insanity were generally regarded as bodily illnesses not differing in any fundamental ways from other diseases." Even the famous psychiatrist Karl Menninger hypothesized in 1922 that schizophrenia was "in most instances the byproduct of viral encephalitis." And although it seems counterintuitive to suggest that humans can catch depression or schizophrenia in the same way we catch the flu, this hypothesis springs from germ theory, developed by Louis Pasteur in the 1860s and Robert Koch in the 1870s, which posits that specific microbes such as bacteria, viruses, and prions (infectious proteins) cause illness.[6]

Although most people think only of physical illness, not mental disease, when they think of germ theory, pioneering psychiatrists like E. Fuller Torrey, the executive director of the Stanley Medical Research Institute (SMRI), have sought to change this. Torrey has long rejected the relegation of mental disease to psychological causes alone and has spent the last half a century tracing the relationship between infection and mental illness.

In the 1990s, Torrey observed that in the late nineteenth century, schizophrenia and bipolar disorder went from being rare diseases to relatively common ones. During the same period he noticed that owning cats as pets replaced regarding them as Satan's minions, relegating them to barns for rodent control, and burning them to celebrate important holidays.

Around the time that England's first cat show was held at the Crystal Palace, in 1871, cat ownership became popular in America. That same year brought a sharp rise in U.S. schizophrenia rates[7] (except among rural Hutterites, who "almost never" keep cats as pets). Cats carry a zoonotic infection (a disease humans acquire from animals) that causes schizophrenia.

In this case, Torrey suspected *Toxoplasma gondii*, an infectious single-celled organism discovered in 1908 by Charles Nicolle and Louis Manceaux of Paris's Institut Pasteur. The parasite lives in the tissues of many warm-blooded animals, but it can reproduce only within the stomachs of felids (domestic cats and other members of the family Felidae), making its survival dependent on access to cats. Most healthy adults are unaffected or only mildly sickened by a *T. gondii* infection, but it produces a variety of serious ailments, including toxoplasmosis, in those

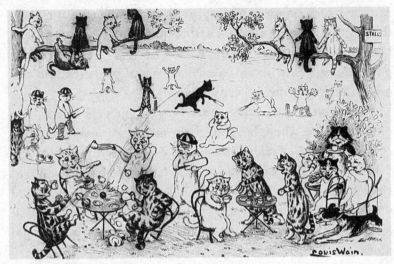

Successful Victorian English artist Louis Wain (1860–1939) was best known for his drawings, which featured large-eyed anthropomorphized cats. Wain spent his last years in a mental hospital where he had been diagnosed with schizophrenia and his images have been used in psychiatric textbooks to document the supposed deterioration of his art as his mental health worsened.

with compromised immune systems and in young children with immature immune defenses.

Torrey and his frequent research partner Robert Yolken of Johns Hopkins University have investigated the roles of influenza, *T. gondii*, and other pathogens in mental disorders. They undertook this research nearly a half century ago, when Freudian and psychosocial paradigms defined mental illness. As the next chapter explains, their efforts helped to shift this paradigm.

A microbial revolution

In his landmark book *The Structure of Scientific Revolutions*, Thomas Kuhn explains that those in the humanities—people who study, for example, eighteenth-century English literature, African American history, or German existentialism—are free to select the most convincing perspectives, assumptions, and causal frameworks within which to interpret their facts, but scientists are bound by a shared overarching theory. Kuhn defines that worldview, or *Weltanschauung,* as "what members of a scientific community, and they alone, share."

A paradigm shift is a revolution, for it seeks to overturn the prevailing worldview. But such an overturning is not to be undertaken lightly, because the scientific community's work, careers, and economies rest on the existing paradigm, and to nullify it is to cross the Rubicon, forever abandoning the rules that had previously defined scientific thought. Having embraced the theory of evolution, scientists cannot return to creationist myths to explain the variety of animal life. Having embraced germ theory, scientists cannot revert to believing that sin, demons, or wandering wombs cause madness or that malarious airs increase one's risk of contracting malaria. We are stuck, as it were, with what we know.

So we must choose our revolutions carefully. Yet the one this book describes—the recognition of infection as an important cause of mental illness—may have already begun; most of us just haven't realized it yet.

I say this because revolution takes place when anomalies arise that the existing worldview cannot explain. For example, it is hard to think of schizophrenia as a genetic disease when genetically identical twins are discordant—that is, when only one of the duo becomes schizophrenic. Such an anomaly doesn't immediately trigger researchers to discard the theory; in fact, many such anomalies are tolerated (or ignored) until a sort of critical mass accumulates that throws the field into "a state of crisis," according to Kuhn. New theories are then proposed, although sometimes they are not really new but ideas that have periodically resurfaced, been marginalized, decried as heresy, and forgotten. The hypothesis that infection causes or encourages common mental illnesses—and some uncommon ones—is an example, because as potential paradigm shifts go, it is a perennial. As I noted above, the theory has been with us since ancient times and reappears intermittently as part of the Western medical paradigm.

No one is suggesting that infection should completely replace stress, genetics, and psychological trauma as an explanation for mental illness, just that infection complements them and joins them as an important causative factor. And it is sometimes the primary factor.

The idea that a case of the flu might consign one to madness sounds fanciful. But consider that we are just now discerning the infectious roots of old familiar physical illnesses, many of which had been supposed to have psychological or behavioral triggers.

Cervical cancer, for example, was long ascribed to sexual immoderation in women and poor hygiene in their male partners, but it is now known to be the legacy of infection by strains of the human papillomavirus, HPV. Ninety percent of ulcers, which were once blamed on a spicy diet and uncontrolled stress, are now known to be caused by *Helicobacter pylori*. Contrary to the theory that held sway as late as the 1990s, heart disease is not a product of having a tense, hostile, angry type A personality but, often, of infection by bacteria including *Streptococcus tigurinus* and *Chlamydophila pneumoniae*.

Bacteria, viruses, parasites, fungi, and the infectious proteins called prions are surfacing as possible causes of mental illness as well, a theory that explains many previously mysterious anomalies. Schizophrenia, for example, has been traced to waves of influenza epidemics as well as to infections with bornavirus; species of adolescent anorexia and Tourette's syndrome have been connected to streptococcal infections that affect the basal ganglia; and autism is linked to marauding infections from children's own guts. This book explores the evidence for all of these and more.

Cartesian skirmishes

In the seventeenth century, René Descartes posited the existence of two fundamental kinds of substance: mental and material.[8] According to this Cartesian dualism, the mental has no spatial existence, and the material cannot think. Substance dualism became popular among scientists and clerics alike, perhaps because it does not preclude the religious belief that immortal souls occupy an independent realm of existence distinct from that of the physical world.[9]

But dualism is far more than a philosophy in medicine; it has long been a political stance as well, adopted as the default position that legitimized and laid a scientific veneer over the struggle of physicians to dominate medical care. Based in part on this theory of dualism, physicians were able to gradually appropriate the care of the physically ill from the clergy, who had established the religious hospitals that had originally assumed the care of the sick.

Still, although the law often required at least one resident physician in a psychiatric hospital or asylum, during the centuries before the discovery of effective medication, doctors were content to leave the care of the mentally ill to the clergy and nuns. However, the majority of the mentally ill were not confined to institutions. Michel Foucault has observed that madmen were allowed to roam freely in medieval Europe and temporarily confined only when their behavior became extreme enough to pose a threat. Moreover, such confinement was long the prerogative of the family, not the doctor. "From the seventeenth century to the nineteenth century, the right to demand the confinement of a madman belonged to the family: it was the family, first of all, that excluded madmen."[10]

But with the eighteenth-century advent of the industrial age, tolerance of the freewheeling idleness of the mad ceased. In 1800, there were only three thousand insane people confined in state-run and religious institutions in all of England. By the end of the century, that number had ballooned to a hundred thousand, and psychiatrists, after gaining experience in the insane asylums, could claim to be experts on madness. In his book *Mind-Forg'd Manacles*, medical historian Roy Porter describes the events leading up to this critical transitional period and, in particular, the changes in the way insanity was perceived.[11]

In France and England, the mad were now incarcerated, but not without company. "They shared their confinement with the unemployed, sick people, old people, all those who were unable to work,"[12] observed Foucault. Later, Freud seemed to reinforce the notion of idleness as a key component of madness when he described the mentally ill patient as "a person who could neither work nor love."[13] The fight for dominance between religious orders and physicians now had an objective: control of the asylums. Physicians vied for the "ownership" of madness, the last major province of health care where treatment was still in the hands of nonphysicians—notably the clergy, whose acknowledged realm was the care of the soul.

The very fact that separate facilities were controlled by separate professions went a long way toward convincing people that the care of the mentally ill was fundamentally different from that of the physically sick. Physicians reinforced this dualism by their insistence on "scientific" causes and models for physical illness. But they had only the naked eye and simple tools like microscopes to rely on—none of the blood assays, electron microscopes, MRIs, or CT scans that reveal pathology to us today. As a result, myopia reigned, as anyone could plainly see that autopsies of the mentally ill did not reveal the trademark anatomical findings, deterioration, or injury that one saw in physical illnesses. Moreover, the heroics of eighteenth-century medicine against physical illness—cupping, bleeding, and purging—had no discernible effect on madness.

By the late eighteenth century, insanity, or "wrongheaded-ness," was regarded by physicians, clergy, and laypersons alike as fundamentally different from corporeal diseases. This schism owed much to Cartesian dualism, but it was heavily reinforced by political events that dealt the prestige of physicians a series of high-profile blows, raising questions about their ability to treat, or even recognize, mental illness.

The mad king

Chief among these events was the madness of King George, against which conventional medical practitioners seemed powerless. In 1765, George III of England, twenty-five, began to complain of an intolerable burning in his limbs and joints. His courtiers had complaints too; they found that he had suddenly become a crashing bore, collaring and speaking without pause or discernible point about hunting, his horses, and the minutiae of English government to anyone he could find. One could not exactly walk out on a garrulous king of England, no matter how narcotic his monologues, so his physicians listened. One of them actually began counting the words in the king's long, meandering sentences, perhaps to ease the ennui. He found that each contained as many as four hundred words, rapidly spoken and tumbling together in the kind of pressured speech that usually signals urgency. The king, however, was in no hurry. He rambled repetitiously for hours on end before becoming agitated and confused, sometimes foaming at the mouth or going into convulsions. His alarmed physicians regularly huddled around him to study the royal signs and symptoms—profuse sweating, intermittent nausea, and a fast pulse—but they were clearly at sea and arrived at no diagnosis. The puzzling speech changes were similar to those of people with mania and malignant euphoria, but his physicians failed to recognize this. They resorted to commonly used measures like blistering George's skin and dosing him with arsenic, a poisonous metalloid so toxic that it remains a commonplace device in murder mysteries. Some now think it worsened George's state. Even after the king's urine turned blue, the court physicians proved unable to render a diagnosis, to say nothing of a cure.

It fell to a clergyman named Francis Willis to heal him. After undergraduate studies at Oxford, Willis was ordained an Anglican priest and given a fellowship at his alma mater in 1740. In 1776 he moved to Greatford Hall in Lincolnshire and transformed it into a unique private sanatorium. In contrast to the prisonlike asylums of his day, Willis's treatment facility went beyond restraints and straitjackets and focused on compassion, cheerfulness, industry, fresh air, and exercise. His prime tenet was respect for individual dignity; he ignored class distinctions and insisted on neatness of dress. Strangers were often astonished by the sight of humble Greatford residents—mentally ill gardeners, plowmen, and other laborers—strolling the grounds dressed like the London gentlemen among them, in silk waistcoats and breeches, powdered wigs and white stockings. Willis's success in curing titled Englishmen caught the attention of George's deeply concerned wife, Queen Charlotte, who brought Willis to court in 1788.

Francis Willis arrived at court, seemingly the perfect man for the job. Not only could he boast a dramatic string of successes in treating the mentally ill, but he also possessed an unusual attribute for a minister—a medical degree, if not membership in the medical fraternity.

King George's doctors refused to accept him as a professional peer and referred to him as "nothing more than a mountebank." Nor did English medical society in general respect his credentials; for example, he was never admitted to the Royal College of Physicians.

There may have been good reason. Early in his career, as he pursued his unusual mental-health treatments, Willis had represented himself as a physician and practiced medicine without a degree. In 1759, concerned about possible legal consequences, he induced friends at Oxford to grant him a medical degree after the fact and without the usual training—a physician in name only.[14]

Court physicians were inclined to forgive none of this—the specious medical degree, the iconoclastic methods, and, perhaps worst of all, Willis's success. They clamored against Willis's appointment, but Queen Charlotte and the English government were desperate for a cure and held firm because the king's illness was proving disastrous. Some blamed it for the poor political judgment the king was exercising, including the vengeful iron hand he took with the American colonies that resulted in England's humiliating defeat in the 1776 War of Independence.

Unlike the court physicians, who had offered jargon-laden explanations to the queen as they tried one unsuccessful remedy after another, Willis explained his methods in simple, accessible terms and with a warm, respectful manner. Under Willis's care, the king was made to take fresh air and regular exercise and to pay careful attention to his grooming. Willis spoke with and sometimes lectured the king with compassion and consideration. But Willis was practical as well. He was not above restraining the king and locking him in a room in Greatford when he thought it necessary to avoid flight or self-harm.

I cannot find evidence that Willis made a definitive diagnosis, but on February 26, 1789, Willis's bulletin described the "entire cessation of his Majesty's illness." George was cured, to the nation's relief, and the Reverend Francis Willis was rewarded with an annuity of one thousand pounds, state portraits, and a special commemoration medal. He also earned national fame and became so successful that he opened a second asylum at Shillingthorpe Hall. Willis's religious and moral methods of treating mental illness had triumphed where conventional medicine had failed.

However, the still-unnamed disease flared up occasionally, and the king gradually worsened; he spent his final decade straitjacketed and hidden away in Windsor Castle, blind, his insanity interspersed with tragic periods of lucidity. He finally died, in 1802, to be remembered as the mad king who lost America.

Postmortem diagnosis is a popular hobby, and most think that George III suffered from the genetic disease porphyria, whose name comes from the Greek word *porphyrus*, meaning "purple," because royally hued excreta are hallmarks of the disease. Porphyria is often inherited, which bolsters the belief that it was George's ailment, because it afflicted his son George IV; his granddaughter Princess Charlotte, who died during childbirth of complications of the disease;[15] and other relatives of his, including Mary, Queen of Scots, and her son, King James I of England.

It wasn't until 1871, more than a century after King George fell ill, that Felix Hoppe-Seyler determined the mechanism by which porphyria develops. Various signs and symptoms accompany the eight known types of porphyria,[16] but they all involve the abnormal accumulation of porphyrins or their precursors. These compounds are required for heme production, an essential component of blood and cellular metabolism, but porphyrins are toxic when they accumulate, causing symptoms where they build up.[17]

The most common physical signs and symptoms include severe, burning abdominal pain, bluish to reddish urine, leg and arm paralysis or weakness, a rapid pulse, and hypertension.

But they also include psychological changes such as anxiety, irritability, and confusion that can progress to depression or delirium if porphyrins hamper neural transmission.

The inability of King George's physicians, presumably the best in the nation, to diagnose and treat the king's lunacy dealt a staggering blow to the profession, undermining faith in medical doctors' fitness to care for the mentally ill. And the success of the Reverend Willis seemed to validate the clergy's primacy in dealing with emotional woes. The madness of King George also contributed to the schism between physical and mental illness by supporting the assumption that if physicians couldn't effectively treat mental illness, it must not be physical.

Even today, the case of King George remains controversial, and doctors fail to agree on his diagnosis. Some theorize that George's blue urine was a red herring, a side effect of the deep blue gentian flowers with which his doctors dosed him. Some are convinced that his madness was iatrogenic—that is, that he was poisoned by the arsenic used to treat him. Writing in the journal *History of Psychiatry,* Timothy J. Peters and Allan Beveridge make a strong case for bipolar disorder.[18]

But whether porphyria was the right diagnosis or not, most pertinent to this discussion is the fact that the ailment is neither strictly a mental disorder nor strictly a physical one; it is both. George's physicians erred when they focused on the physical signs and symptoms of his illness and refused to see that any treatment must also address the disease's heavy psychological freight, from anxiety to confusion and delirium. This myopia persists today. Given the tools and medications doctors had at the time, understanding the psychological component of George's illness might not have helped physicians treat the king, but insisting on viewing a disease as mental *or* physical when indeed it was both obscured its true nature and may have obscured potential treatments as well.

The false dichotomy of mental versus physical disease was further reinforced by infamous cases of medical abuse and neglect that were addressed by clergy and social workers. For example, in 1790, Quaker Hannah Mills, a melancholic widow from Leeds, England, was brought to the York lunatic asylum. The institution prohibited all visits from her family and friends, and although Hannah was young and physically healthy, she died there just six weeks after arriving, under suspicious circumstances. Fellow Quaker William Tuke of York was appalled to hear of her fate, and he later learned that the asylum's inmates were restrained inhumanely and warehoused in squalid conditions. The "therapeutic" emphasis of the lunatic asylum seemed to fall on controlling and quieting the human mass. Tuke was determined to create a humane treatment center utilizing Christian precepts and ethics, a facility where he could employ psychologically based approaches that came to be known as *moral treatment*. He raised funds and consulted his religious brethren before building the York Retreat, which proved instrumental in the development of more humane methods in the custody and care of people with mental disorders.

Tuke's clean, attractive, dignified facilities and caring staff helped the patients weather psychological issues. So did the retreat's welcoming of visits from family, and the Tuke center became a world-famous institution, heading a successful revolution in the care and treatment of the mentally ill.[19]

The York Retreat's philosophy, like that of Francis Willis, focused on the psychological rather than the physical cause of mental illness. It helped establish madness as distinct from the body and best treated by the religious orders. In this era, when medicine could offer little for serious physical illnesses besides supportive care or ill-advised heroics, hospitals in general were unpopular destinations. Invidious comparisons between the supportive treatment offered by the Quakers and the medical hellholes where patients rarely improved further undermined faith in medical doctors' ability to understand and care for the mentally ill.

Who would rule the asylum—doctors or religious orders?

Rush to medical judgment

Doctors like Benjamin Rush[20] sought to appropriate the care of mentally ill patients by ascribing their illnesses to purely physical causes, such as infection.

Benjamin Rush, revered as the "father of American psychiatry," knew that doctors and clergy were in contention for the control of mental-health care. And Rush, a signer of the Declaration of Independence, was a fighter; he was a surgeon with the Philadelphia militia when they battled the British, and he won appointment as surgeon general of the middle department of the Continental army.

Admittedly, the battles he chose to fight could be quixotic or downright reckless and reactionary, as when he insisted on practicing bloodletting years after it had been proven not only useless but dangerous.[21] He also freely administered mercury even though its toxic effects were well known. Rush was a vocal and militant abolitionist and one of the few white doctors of the era who championed black medical aspirants, but he sabotaged his fine antislavery sentiments and writings when he purchased a slave, William Grubber, in 1776, whom he retained even after joining the Pennsylvania Abolition Society in 1784.

In his fight for the prestige and primacy of American physicians, Rush insisted that the fundamental pathology of diseases of the mind was wholly somatic, lying within "the blood vessels of the brain." In his 1812 psychiatry text *Medical Inquiries and Observations upon the Diseases of the Mind,* Rush included the first detailed taxonomy of mental disorders, each with its own physical cause. He cited disruptions of blood circulation and sensory overload as the basis of mental illness, and he treated his patients with devices meant to improve circulation to the brain, including such Rube Goldberg designs as a centrifugal spinning board and a restraining chair with a head enclosure.

Rush, whose image adorns the seal of the American Psychiatric Association today, tended to find physical causes, including infectious ones, for many human conditions. For example, in 1792 he theorized that the dark skin of African Americans was caused by a form of leprosy, predicting that with proper treatment, blacks could be "cured" and become white.[22]

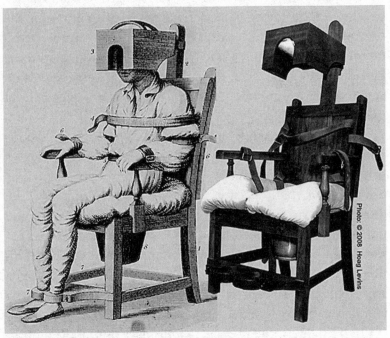

Dr. Benjamin Rush designed two mechanical contrivances to aid in the treatment of the insane. The belief at the time was that "madness" was an arterial disease, an inflammation of the brain. Pictured here is the "tranquilizing chair" in which patients were confined. The chair was supposed to control the flow of blood toward the brain and, by lessening muscular action or reducing motor activity, reduce the force and frequency of the pulse. Both of Rush's devices were supposed to exert an influence in some way on circulation, which was believed to be essential to the successful treatment of the insane. In actuality, they did neither harm nor good.

In 1812, the politically powerful Rush led the successful charge to establish doctors' primacy over the asylum. He did so in part by ascribing physical causes to mental illnesses, and over the next few decades, new research supported his claims. Wilhelm Griesinger's 1845 book *Psychische Krankheiten sind Erkrankungen des Gehirns* (*Mental Diseases Are Diseases of the Brain*) convinced German physicians, generally acknowledged to be the world's best, that mental diseases had physical origins. Still, some physicians remained skeptical. After all, changes in the "sick" brain could not be seen with the naked eye or a microscope. The evidence was thin.

Until one disorder changed everything.

Unmasking a familiar madness

Paresis is a forgotten word, but it was once a familiar species of madness. The diagnosis was given to one of every five inmates of New York City's mental asylums by the 1920s[23] and it was twice as common in Europe; Robert Schumann, Guy de Maupassant, Gaetano Donizetti, and Friedrich Nietzsche number among its victims.[24] Some speculate, with less compelling data, that it also killed Hitler and Christopher Columbus.[25] Also known as dementia paralytica and as general paresis of the insane, the condition was first described in 1822 by physician Antoine-Laurent Bayle. He noted that paretics, as they were called, experienced a coarsening of the personality followed by mania, vivid delusions, and dementia. After a period of months to years, this psychological deterioration culminated in a "rapid and complete mental decay" that included frequent seizures, paralysis, incontinence, psychosis, severe visual disturbances, and death.

For seventy years after Bayle described the disorder, doctors attributed this common mental malady to the usual suspects — trauma, overwork, anxiety, and even intemperance — because paresis, like many a mental disorder before it, was viewed as a punishment for depravity.

In 1857, Drs. Johannes Friedrich Esmark and W. Jessen suggested a biological cause for paresis: syphilis. To bolster their case they compiled copious statistics on paresis patients who also suffered from syphilis, and they reported their findings widely. Intrigued, other researchers began to correlate paresis with patients' medical histories and found that a history of syphilis was extremely common. Moreover, Wassermann tests later developed to detect syphilis quantified the high correlation of syphilis in paretics by confirming that the spirochete bacteria *Treponema pallidum* lurked within their brains. Many researchers started to view paresis as the tertiary stage of syphilis, which often attacked the brain indiscriminately, and they began referring to it as neurosyphilis. This theory held out hope that if syphilis was ever cured, paresis could be too.

Nineteenth-century asylum keepers, however, persisted in viewing paresis as wholly mental in character. The long-standing insistence on divorcing physical illnesses from mental ones had to do with religious philosophy and culture but also with the politics of the asylum, which remained a battleground between physicians and religious and philosophical healers.[26]

Matters were complicated by the fact that most physicians, despite the evidence that paresis was the mental manifestation of a physical disease, continued to treat paretics with the same ineffectual therapeutics given other mentally ill patients. Traditional treatments such as "douches, cold packs, mercury, blistering of the scalp, venesection, leeching, sexual abstinence, and holes drilled into the skull [trephination]" continued—without positive results. Even when toxic mercury-based treatments for syphilis were replaced by Paul Ehrlich's safer, more effective arsenic-based Salvarsan (also called arsphenamine and compound 606), it was not used against paresis.

But in June 1917, Professor Julius Wagner-Jauregg of the

University of Vienna Hospital for Nervous and Mental Diseases undertook a radical approach. He had noticed that some paretic patients improved markedly after contracting an infectious illness that gave them fevers. He decided to fight fire with fire by turning one disease against another: he sought to suppress the symptoms of paresis by infecting its sufferers with malaria.

Wagner-Jauregg reasoned that the infamous high fevers of malaria might kill the syphilis spirochetes, or at least inactivate them, because many bacteria can operate only within a very narrow temperature range. This is why our bodies respond to many infectious diseases with fever. Wagner-Jauregg hoped that malarial fevers would raise the paretics' body heat above the spirochetes' survival zone, rendering them unable to do further harm.

He inoculated Austrian subjects with malaria-infected blood and was rewarded with fevers that soared to 106 degrees F. In the end, Wagner-Jauregg recorded dramatic clinical improvements, if no cures.[27] The world was so gratified by the apparent success of malaria therapy that Wagner-Jauregg won the Nobel Prize in Physiology or Medicine in 1927.[28] This despite the fact that the treatment proved dangerous—as many as 15 percent of the subjects died—and that his studies did not use any modern techniques for minimizing bias.[29] As a result, his skewed conclusions reflected what he wished to see—that malaria therapy helped paresis patients. Wagner-Jauregg offered evidence, rather than proof, to substantiate the theory that infection causes paresis, and that evidence was not free of bias. But it—and the Nobel Prize—made powerful arguments for infection.

One might think that Wagner-Jauregg's Nobel Prize–winning studies of this common mental disease would help elevate biological psychiatry. But by the 1930s, Wagner-Jauregg's work was eclipsed by his compatriot and fellow neurologist Sigmund Freud.

Freud, the founder of psychoanalysis, began his career studying microscopic neuroanatomy at Vienna General Hospital, dissecting the nerves of crayfish and investigating cerebral palsy. But brain science was so primitive in the late nineteenth century that the basic workings of the neuron were a mystery, and Freud left objective physiologic science behind, choosing instead to study the mind's role in repressing drives that are "powerful enough to evoke madness" when neglected.[30] To combat such repression, Freud refined the "talking cure," or the practice of psychoanalysis, in which doctors perceive and interpret the unconscious struggles of patients as a means of helping them to achieve greater self-awareness.

Freud's conception of mental illness as arising from psychic conflicts resonated with mental-health providers and their patients, much more so than the biophysiological, infection-related model did, and the psychoanalytical approach transformed twentieth-century psychiatry. Upstaging the infectious nature of paresis, Freudian psychoanalysis swept aside the startling role of infection in mental illness[31] and reinforced the divide between mental and physical illness.

Under the auspices of the Rockefeller Foundation, Mark Boyd became one of many researchers who sought to reproduce Wagner-Jauregg's celebrated successes. But this research also lacked some of today's controls against researcher bias. Double-blind studies and other techniques that we currently rely on to reduce bias in study interpretation were not in common use in that era, and these experiments were repeated throughout the first half of the twentieth century with the same lack of rigor. So once again, it was all too easy for researchers to see what they wished to see—that their paresis patients were being helped by infection with a chronic, debilitating disease.

But there still was no cure for syphilis—which meant there was none for paresis. Because demonstrating the infectious nature of paresis did not appreciably change the way doctors treated it, the discovery did not improve the clinical course of the disease. What's more, associating paresis with syphilis added the stigma of venereal disease to that of insanity. As historian Allan M. Brandt noted in his masterly *No Magic Bullet,* "Venereal disease remained a symptom of social decay and sexual evil," and psychiatrist Joel T. Braslow observed that "newspaper and magazine articles in periodicals such as the *New York Times, Good Housekeeping, Scientific American, Hygeia, Reader's Digest, Newsweek,* and *Popular Mechanics* depicted neurosyphilitics in highly value-laden, moralistic terms," using phrases such as "'wretched maniacs,' 'those whose sins it rewarded,' and 'doomed human derelicts.'"[32]

Inspired by Wagner-Jauregg's Nobel and buoyed by the clinical benefits touted in parallel studies, researchers continued with malaria-therapy experiments until 1943, the year when a portentous paper by John F. Mahoney[33] demonstrated that penicillin cured syphilis. The antibiotic arrested paresis too, proving that the mental illness was indeed a late stage of syphilis infection. As physicians wielded penicillin against paresis, it all but vanished from the United States, and today, you'd have to visit a developing nation with poor health care to find a case.

The question of malaria therapy's effectiveness became clinically moot, at least against paresis in the West, but the enigmatic prospect of using one disease to fight another lingers as an unanswered question of medical history.

Germ theory: a paradigm shift

Before Wagner-Jauregg won the Nobel and Freud forged the future of psychiatry, a paradigm shift had already taken place that transformed science's approach to the nature of disease. It is the very framework that supports the role of infection in mental illness—germ theory. Developed by Louis Pasteur and Robert Koch, germ theory posits that specific microbes such as bacteria, viruses, and prions (infectious proteins) cause illness.[34]

Although nineteenth-century German bacteriologists Robert Koch and Friedrich Loeffler were the first to provide evidence that infinitesimally small life-forms called microbes caused disease, scientists as early as the seventeenth century had suggested that tiny beings might be the source of illness. They could produce no credible proof, however, and it was not until 1883 that the microscope revealed the pathogens, disproving theories that illness was caused by sinful behaviors or poisonous vapors.

Germ theory—the discovery of these tiny agents of infection—accelerated treatment and prevention. Pasteur saved the lives of millions of women[35] when he discovered the cause of childbed fever. Germ theory also revealed to him that bacteria were the source of wine spoilage and he figured out how to prevent it through a process we still call pasteurization—heating the libations to kill bacteria, a deeply appreciated feat in oenophile France. For his part, Koch discovered that the airborne *Mycobacterium tuberculosis* caused the dreaded tuberculosis and that *Bacillus anthracis* caused anthrax. As a result of these findings, infectious agents were widely acknowledged as a cause of disease that had previously been ascribed to vague "miasmas" and "air."

By the twentieth century the paradigm shift to germ theory had changed the face of medicine. The most common, terrifying killers, including tuberculosis, smallpox, influenza, diphtheria, yellow fever, bubonic plague, and whooping cough, were now known to result from infection by pathogens. Accordingly, scientists turned their attention to devising vaccines, antibiotics, and public-health measures to stem their spread. The smallpox virus was eradicated, except for some samples preserved in Western laboratories. As medical innovations tamed these illnesses, Americans began living longer and eventually dying of other illnesses like cancers and heart disease (although we now recognize many of these diseases as infectious in origin as well).

But the germ-theory paradigm shift bypassed mental illness. Paresis was recognized as infectious and then rooted out of the asylum by penicillin, but diseases like schizophrenia, depression, bipolar disorder, and obsessive-compulsive disorder remained the province of mental health, with its emphasis on talk therapy, behavioral conditioning, cognitive therapy, and other manipulations of the mind. By the 1980s new medications based on altering brain chemistry tacitly acknowledged the physical nature of much mental illness, but the supposed dichotomy between physical and mental illness stubbornly remained and still does to this day. Thus it is that even in our time, when most psychiatrists treat only with medication, the growing evidence that infection makes a strong contribution to mental illness is studiously avoided.

This book makes the case for ending that avoidance. In the chapters that follow, I will discuss the evidence that influenza as well as the parasite *Toxoplasma gondii* are implicated in schizophrenia and von Economo's encephalitis. I'll talk about how Group A streptococci can cause anorexia, obsessive-compulsive disorder, and Tourette's syndrome and how microbes residing in our guts cause some cases of autism as well as various autoimmune diseases with psychiatric components. I'll look at how prions, or infectious proteins, cause Creutzfeldt-Jakob disease, or CJD, the human version of mad cow disease, which is marked by personality changes, depression, memory loss, and impaired thinking as well as movement disorders.[36] I'll explore how rare complications of measles and some forms of food poisoning engender mental derangement serious enough to require institutionalization. Certainly infection is unlikely to stand alone as a cause in many ailments, as it does for paresis; the traditional risk factors of genetics, stress, and other environmental pressures are sure to apply as well. Yet most researchers into the infection connection estimate that known pathogens account for 10 to 20 percent of cases of mental illness.

Paresis is not the only precedent. Belief in the infectious roots of madness is not an exclusively postmodern view; in fact, a few mental illnesses have long been recognized as infectious. Rabies immediately comes to mind. Caused by one of the lyssaviruses, named after Lyssa, the Greek goddess of madness and rage, the disease is a ferociously aggressive mental state caused by the bite of an infected animal—or human. Ergotism is another example: ergot, fungi that infect rye, produces the alkaloid ergotamine, which causes burning sensations, tissue loss, psychosis, hallucinations, irrational behavior, seizures, convulsions, and even death. Eating bread or other foods made with tainted rye has been recognized as a cause of dramatic syndromes such as St. Anthony's fire during the medieval period and the Great Fear in France.[37] Some have ascribed the mass hysteria of the Salem witch trials to ergotism, although others dispute that theory.[38]

Despite this, our authoritative references still maintain the ironclad distinction between mental and physical disease. Editors of the *Diagnostic and Statistical Manual of Mental Disorders,* known as the *DSM,* admit that the text has reinforced the strict but often imaginary dichotomy between mental and physical disease. "The term 'mental disorder' unfortunately implies a distinction between 'mental disorders' and 'physical disorders' that is a reductionist anachronism of mind/body dualism," the (now superseded) *DSM-IV* website notes, adding that "the term persists…because we have not found an appropriate substitute."[39]

Still, the very word *mental* in *mental disorders* seems to contradict the idea of a biomedical basis for these conditions, even though some consciousness research in neuroscience has emerged with evidence for just such biological underpinnings. Writing in *Neuroscience,* Chun Siong Soon and his team found that "in some contexts, the decisions that a person makes can be detected up to 10 seconds in advance by means of scanning their brain activity."[40] Furthermore, subjective experiences and covert attitudes are observable, providing[41] "strong empirical evidence that cognitive processes have physical basis in the brain,[42] although it does not completely dispel the possibility of mind-body distinction."

The price of revolution

Maybe it shouldn't surprise us that mental-health professionals continue to behave as though the mind/body divide were real. One survey found that physicians think of mental illness as a continuum, from the physiological disorders, such as autism, to the nonbiological disorders, such as adjustment disorder.[43] Respondents said they believed medication was the best treatment for the more biological diseases and talk therapy was best for the nonbiological disorders.

The problem lies in whether these same doctors actually understand which mental disorders are biological and which are not. Writing in the *Wilson Quarterly,* psychological anthropologist Tanya Luhrmann of Stanford describes the Research Domain Criteria, a project that proposes to dispense with the diagnoses enshrined in the *Diagnostic and Statistical Manual of Mental Disorders* and elsewhere. It instead seeks to address the specific challenges and issues facing individual patients, from sadness to phobias to memory loss. But, she writes, there is too much at stake economically for this plan to go into effect, because the payment system depends on "the fiction of clear-cut, biologically distinct diseases."[44]

She's right. Economics is an important factor in any element of U.S. medicine. But there's even more at stake here, because, as Thomas Kuhn reminds us, scientists' bodies of work, careers, livelihoods, and prestige rest on the existing paradigm, so toppling it can be a very risky and difficult enterprise. Resistance is natural, making revolution painful and costly in terms of far more than money.

Yet, as research gains in sophistication and medical knowledge increases, so do examples of how permeable the diaphanous membrane is between sickness of the mind and ailments of the body.

We know, for example, that infection profoundly changes a sick person's behavior in a predictable manner. We can see this very easily in the elderly whose immune systems have lost their vigor. When my mother was confined to a nursing home with dementia, she had lost the ability to walk, initiate speech, or do any but the simplest tasks, but she smiled alertly, nodded meaningfully, and understood much of what was said to her. We had many conversations without her saying a word other than *good* or *yes*. But whenever she became listless, unengaged, and uncommunicative, failing to eat and interact with others, I would suspect an infection, and I soon learned that other families in her nursing home saw the same dynamic with their loved ones.

The nurses tended to validate our hunches. In fact, the positive screens sometimes seemed a formality, verifying the infection that everyone already suspected based on the elder's sick behavior. Of course, many factors can be involved, but behavioral changes in response to an infection are not confined to people with paresis or the elderly. Whether you tend to be reclusive, gregarious, or somewhere in between, your behavior hews closely to a new norm when you are stricken with, say, the flu, as Martin H. Fischer, MD, hinted when he quipped, "When a man lacks mental balance in pneumonia he is said to be delirious. When he lacks mental balance without the pneumonia, he is pronounced insane by all smart doctors."

We see the same overlapping of the physical and the mental in established mental diseases caused by physical infections, like paresis and rabies, but also in novel infections that lead to more familiar diseases, like depression and schizophrenia.

The threat may begin in the womb, as the next chapter reveals.

CHAPTER 2

The Fetus as Battleground: Early Exposure and Psychiatric Fate

Our mothers' wombs the tiring-houses be,
where we are dressed for this short comedy.

— SIR WALTER RALEIGH

In the early autumn of 1957, Edwin Fuller Torrey, a premedical student at Princeton, got a phone call from his worried mother. His sister, Rhoda, seventeen, an excellent student and popular cheerleader who was heading to Elmira College herself in a week, had begun behaving bizarrely. Just then, she was hallucinating. Lying on the lawn of their family's home in Clinton, New York, her eyes fixed on a spectacle that only she could see, Rhoda repeatedly shouted, "The British are coming! The British are coming!"[1]

"We knew nothing about what was going on because people don't grow up knowing about these diseases, especially in the 1950s," recalls Torrey. To find answers and treatment, Torrey, Rhoda, and their mother made a pilgrimage to the revered Massachusetts General Hospital, or MGH, a Harvard-affiliated institution dubbed "Man's Greatest Hospital" by Boston wags. There, doctors told Torrey's mother, a young widow raising her children alone, that Rhoda had schizophrenia caused by "dysfunctional" family relationships. "It's hard to believe now, but the Freudian ideas about schizophrenia were prominent," says Torrey. "My mother was told that my sister got sick because my father had died and because of problems within the family."

Rhoda suffered from schizophrenia for the rest of her life, spending long periods in Marcy State Hospital and Mohawk Valley Psychiatric Hospital before her 2010 death in Utica, New York, at age seventy.

What causes schizophrenia? While its origins are much debated, its ravages are devastatingly clear. Rhoda's story is all too common. Schizophrenia tends to seize the young, as early as the late teens or twenties, just as adolescence begins to yield to the promise of education, career, love, marriage, and a family of one's own. As their peers embark on college, careers, and marriage, the afflicted find themselves suddenly struggling to complete their thoughts, communicate logically, discern the difference between actual events and hallucinations, and perform simple tasks of self-care.

It's hard to say which aspect of schizophrenia is most terrible. The disease brings disorganized thinking; the invention of meaningless words, called *neologisms*; and difficulties in sustaining activities and in speaking to and connecting with others.[2] Plagued by failing executive functioning, some people with schizophrenia find it hard to understand information and use it rationally to make decisions—for example, to prioritize tasks. Others find that they can no longer retain memories well or focus their attention. To rise in the morning, bathe, dress, prepare a meal, or carry on a conversation while hearing voices, hallucinating, and continually losing one's equanimity and train of thought can prove impossible. So can accepting the confusion, delusions, loss of friends, and the feeling of one's very personality slipping away as psychosis and bizarre behaviors take over.

The murky origins of this tragic psychosis escalate the fear it engenders. Many theories seek to explain the alarming symptoms that can accompany schizophrenia, such as the break from reality and aural and visual hallucinations. Dr. Miriam Spering, codirector of the University of British Columbia's NOVA Lab, thinks that the *efference copy* produced by a normal nervous system is key. An efference copy is an internal copy of an outgoing signal that's sent to the motor system. Efference copies let the brain predict what an action's effects will be. When a brain cannot generate or interpret efference copies, the person cannot correct incomplete perceptions. To fill in the blanks, the brain may resort to prior experience. But combining old images with experiences in present time, Spering's theory suggests, can present as hallucinations and other symptoms of psychosis.[3]

In the United States and most of the developed world, medications help many people with schizophrenia, and some of them lead near-normal lives. But few schizophrenics are cured, and only half are treated effectively. There are several reasons for this, but one factor is anosognosia—a lack of awareness of their limitations. Because many people with schizophrenia don't accept that they have an illness or don't understand how serious it is, they fail to take their medications or get treatment. This ensures that they will remain ill.

Schizophrenics are damaged not only by the reality of their symptoms but also by the mythology of the disease. According to the National Alliance on Mental Illness (NAMI), 64 percent of people in the United States think that schizophrenia is characterized by a split personality that makes its sufferers careen between normal and outrageous behavior. This false belief feeds the perception that schizophrenics are volatile and prone to unpredictable violence, which in turn causes society to view them as dangerous elements that must be controlled.

Dr. David Crepaz-Keay, chief of social inclusion at the UK's Mental Health Foundation, agrees: "People with a diagnosis of schizophrenia are feared still and perceived as dangerous."

Crepaz-Keay has personal experience to supplement his expertise: he was diagnosed with schizophrenia in 1979.

Is there a rational basis for the stereotype of the violent schizophrenic? In 2006, Dr. Seena Fazel of Sweden's Karolinska Institute conducted a study that found that only one in twenty crimes is committed by a person with mental illness, a far smaller number than most people assume. Fazel also found that schizophrenics were four times more likely than those without the disorder to commit a violent offense—*if* they also engaged in drug or alcohol abuse. However, the odds fell to nearly normal—only 1.2 times more likely than others to engage in violence—when there was no drug or alcohol abuse involved.

Thus, the violent propensities of the mentally ill are both exaggerated and controllable, says Fazel: "There are evidence-based treatment strategies for drug and alcohol abuse, so the risk of violence can be reduced."

Schizophrenia is just one type of psychosis, a category of mental disease whose hallmark is the inability to distinguish reality from delusions and hallucinations. But it is one of the most common and important psychoses. This chapter's main focus is the evidence that infectious agents drive schizophrenia, but I'll also discuss the infectious roots of some other psychoses, such as the mental disorders that followed in the wake of the 1918 influenza pandemic.

Schizophrenia is most often described as a universal disease that affects between 1 and 2 percent of the global population. The World Health Organization (WHO) reports that twenty-four million people worldwide have it, and half of them get no care. In much of the developing world, with its inadequate public-health infrastructure, that is likely to be a gross underestimate. But the disease also presents in a spectrum of variations, so the abilities of people with schizophrenia vary dramatically, and many navigate the world quite capably despite the disease's hurdles.

The outcomes of schizophrenia also vary dramatically around the globe. Rigorous WHO studies conducted over nearly two decades have revealed that people with schizophrenia in developing countries are far more likely than those in the United States to marry, hold a job, and maintain their social status. Americans with schizophrenia are far more likely than schizophrenics in the Global South (Africa, Central and Latin America, and most of Asia) to commit suicide, while the latter are more likely to recover. Anthropologists and psychiatrists ascribe most of these dramatic differences in outcome to culture rather to biology, although some psychiatrists consider the WHO studies flawed and deny that any such "Third World" advantage exists. This basic disagreement highlights how much remains unknown about this common psychosis.

But our ignorance of what causes schizophrenia may be the most dangerous unknown. Medication can tame its symptoms, but it does so very inconsistently. Not until we understand the cause of the disease can we craft better treatments and devise preventives.

In trying to understand the cause of schizophrenia's mystifying symptoms and patterns, scientists have intensely examined the usual suspects that are perp-walked in the search for the etiology of a mental ailment: psychological experiences, trauma, stress, and—especially—genetics.

The limits of genetics

We often read of genetic studies performed to determine the risk of developing schizophrenia or other mental illnesses, which lends credence to the belief that these diseases are genetic in nature. But the evidence is easily explained by infectious agents as well. In fact, as evolutionary biologist Paul Ewald wrote in *Perspectives in Biological Medicine*: "Although evidence generally accepted as demonstrating genetic causation can be readily explained by hypotheses of infectious causation, some of the evidence implicating infectious causation cannot be similarly explained by genetic causation."[4]

Still, it is easy to see why contemporary psychiatric research focuses largely on genetics. For one thing, schizophrenia does run in families. One of every one hundred U.S. residents has it, but the likelihood of an individual having it leaps tenfold, to one in ten, if an immediate family member is affected. This pattern makes genetics a favored research focus, and to elucidate its role, scientists have conducted genetic research, including twin studies, for decades.

Scientists often investigate the genetic contributions to disease by comparing the medical fates of identical twins—also called monozygotic, or MZ, twins—who have long been assumed to share all their genes. Comparing these twins should rule out genetics as a variable so scientists can concentrate on searching for environmental differences, such as diet, poisoning, trauma, family psychosocial dynamics, or infection. When MZ twins have been subjected to different agents or exposures—because they have been raised in different families or simply because they have had different experiences—comparing them shows how environment might affect risks and offers clues as to why one twin develops schizophrenia when the other does not.

For it is usually the case in schizophrenia that only one twin is affected. If one identical twin develops it, there is only a 40 percent chance that the other will, which means that schizophrenia cannot be wholly genetic. Were genetics the sole determinant, every twin pair would be *concordant*—that is, either both individuals would have schizophrenia or neither would have it.

However, when identical twins are compared to fraternal, or

dizygotic (DZ), twins, who share only half their genes as opposed to all of them, the results suggest the strength of genetics as a contributor to the disease: only 17 percent of fraternal twins are concordant, compared to 40 percent of identical twins.

According to Torrey, now the director of the Stanley Medical Research Institute in Chevy Chase, Maryland, genetics is an important factor in schizophrenia, but a secondary one. "I personally think that the majority of cases of schizophrenia are caused by an infectious agent with a genetic predisposition, and that the initial infection takes place in early childhood," says Torrey. "From two-thirds to three-quarters of schizophrenia cases (as well as cases of schizoaffective and bipolar disorders) will turn out to have an infectious component, although they may have genetic predisposition as well."

Moreover, no single-gene mutation that produces schizophrenia has been identified. This could mean that a complex interaction among genes causes schizophrenia, or it could mean that family members of a schizophrenic have a heightened risk of developing the disease because they share another, nongenetic risk factor, such as exposure to the same toxin or microbe.

People with schizophrenia suffer higher rates of rare genetic mutations, genetic differences that involve hundreds of different genes and may disrupt brain development. So, many genes may interact in a complex multifactorial manner with one another or with an environmental insult—including pathogens—to produce schizophrenia. Thus, genes and microbes are not mutually exclusive causes of the disease. Both may be necessary, and there are likely to be more than one set of factors, just as many genes have been implicated so far.

And while twin studies have provided some of the best-regarded evidence for genetic roots of schizophrenia, they have been haunted by several misconceptions and limitations. For one thing, twins are not truly representative of the population; they're more often born premature and lower in weight than singletons.[5]

As I've said, if schizophrenia were wholly genetic, we would expect a 100 percent concordance. But 52 percent—more than half—of schizophrenic MZ twins are discordant, and so are 40 percent of twin pairs with autism. Yet researchers have tended to see the glass as half full, arguing that a 52 percent discordance rate for schizophrenia means that 48 percent of MZ twins *are* concordant for the disorder, suggesting a strong role for genetics.

The problem is, identical twins are not genetically identical. Although they have the same DNA sequences, identical twins vary slightly genetically for several reasons, from changes called single nucleotide polymorphisms (SNPs) to copy number variations (CNVs), in which small additions or deletions are made to regions of the DNA.[6] DNA methylation, a biochemical process

Pairwise Twin Concordance Rates for Schizophrenia and Other Disorders of the Central Nervous System

Disorder	Identical Twins (%)	Fraternal Twins (%)
Huntington's disease	100 (14/14)	20 (1/5)
Down's syndrome	95 (18/19)	2 (2/127)
Epilepsy	61 (20/46)	10 (13/126)
Mental retardation	60 (18/30)	9 (7 /77)
Bipolar disorder	56 (44/79)	14 (16/111)
Cerebral palsy	40 (6/15)	0 (0/21)
Autism	36 (4/11)	0 (0/10)
Poliomyelitis	36 (5/14)	6 (2/31)
Congenital anomalies of the CNS	33 (2/6)	0 (0/5}
Schizophrenia	28 (97 /341)	6 (36/587)
Multiple sclerosis	27 (17 /62)	2 (2/88)
Parkinson's disease	0 (0/18)	7 (1/14)

Source: E. Fuller Torrey, Ann E. Bowler, Edward H. Taylor, and Irving I. Gottesman. *Schizophrenia and Manic-Depressive Disorder.* New York: Basic Books, 1994.

in which a methyl group (CH_3) is added to certain DNA building blocks, called nucleotides, is another source of change that affected 6 percent to 20 percent of twins in one study.[7]

Quite aside from these small but possibly significant genetic differences, identical twins can look very different and enjoy vastly different states of health. Twin-to-twin transfusion syndrome is a perfect example. In this syndrome, identical twins differ in weight, color, and overall health. In nearly one of three cases, these identical twins differ so significantly that they don't resemble each other. One twin might weigh as much as two pounds more than the other; this twin owes his size to the fact that the twins shared the same placenta (not all identical twins do) and he received the lion's share of the circulating nutrients and oxygen from their mother during fetal development. In fact, these oversize twins are often born so packed with red cells that they look reddish, while the deprived twins are small, pale,

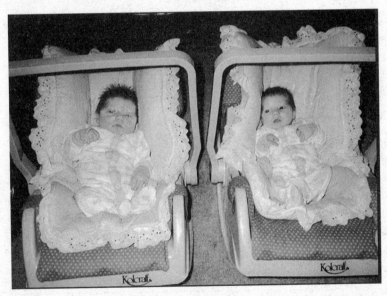

These newborn twins suffer from twin transfusion syndrome (TTS), which causes a marked difference in their size, coloring, and medical status.

with low blood sugar and poorly nourished. The large, ruddy twin is often jaundiced and suffers from cardiac hypertrophy. As you can see from the photograph of twins who have twin-to-twin transfusion syndrome, there is little identical about them aside from their DNA sequences.

The significance for infection and mental illness lies in *why* this dramatic difference defines the twins. Most identical twins— three of every five sets—share a placental circulation, and this circulation carries not only nutrients but also antibodies and pathogens like those suspected of causing schizophrenia— including *Toxoplasma gondii,* influenza, herpes simplex virus 2, cytomegalovirus, and others. This means that identical twins who share a placental circulation[8] risk acquiring these infections and antibodies from their mother. If infection (or damage caused by overzealous antibodies) is the cause of schizophrenia, then twins who share circulations should have a higher percentage of concordance than those who do not.

And this is precisely the case. The late developmental neurobiologist Paul H. Patterson, professor of biological sciences at the California Institute of Technology, performed in-depth studies and determined that "the concordance of schizophrenia in monozygotic twins who share a placenta is much higher (60 percent) than in the minority of monozygotic twins who do not share a placenta (11 percent)."[9] Another 1995 study in the *Schizophrenia Bulletin* analyzed the possible permutations and concluded that "a shared prenatal viral infection may account for much of the high concordance for schizophrenia in identical twins."[10]

It was long thought that a mother's infection could not trigger schizophrenia or other psychoses in the fetus because the placenta acts as a barrier. But, says Torrey, this is a very imperfect barrier and it is frequently breached.[11]

The genetic interplay may be complex, but today, evidence from twin studies and other research suggests that sharing

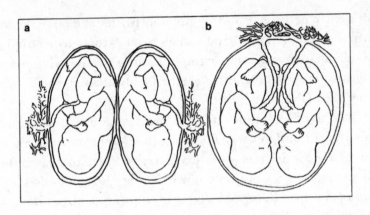

something—infection, nutrition, toxins—in the fetal and early childhood environments increases one's risk of schizophrenia. As this chapter will explain, the evidence for infection's role is now well established.

We know all this today, but over the past half century, doctors have causally linked schizophrenia to everything from family dynamics to brain-chemistry imbalance.

Schizophrenogenic mothers

Not too long ago, in fact, they knew whom to blame: Mom.

"Schizophrenogenic mothers," wrote psychiatrist Frieda Fromm-Reichmann in 1960, trigger insanity in their children with their "domineering, cold, rejecting, possessive, guilt-producing" personalities.[12] Fromm-Reichmann's *Principles of Intensive Psychotherapy* and other textbooks used in psychiatrists' training endorsed these theories, unquestioningly citing bad mothering as a prime risk factor. Throughout the 1980s, schizophrenia continued to be laid at Mom's door as she busily inculcated madness in her children with her harsh, shrewish brand of controlling behavior.

Stanford psychological anthropologist Tanya Luhrmann described the theory behind this maternal vector of insanity in a 2012 essay, explaining, "She delivered conflicting messages of hope and rejection, and her ambivalence drove her child, unable to know what was real, into the paralyzed world of madness. It became standard practice in American psychiatry to regard the mother as the cause of the child's psychosis, and standard practice to treat schizophrenia with psychoanalysis to counteract her grim influence."[13]

Psychiatry held that the fathers in these schizophrenia-incubating homes were abjectly submissive to the mothers—when Dad had not died, absconded, or otherwise disappeared. Thus, fathers could not shield their children from the mothers' poisonous influence. This information was presented unquestioningly in my 1970s psychology classes, and we scribbled away in a Pavlovian response, keeping our heads down and our notebooks filled as we swallowed such "facts" and regurgitated them for tests.

No one understands the corrosive calumny of blaming Mom more than E. F. Torrey, Rhoda's brother. Their mother did not escape the veiled maternal reproach when, on that autumn day in 1957, she and her family sought answers at Massachusetts General Hospital about why schizophrenia had struck Rhoda. "They said it had been brought on by 'family problems' and the shock of my father's death when my sister was young," said Torrey. "It made no more sense to me than the man in the moon. Why didn't *I* have schizophrenia if that's what caused it?"

Torrey researched Rhoda's disease and quickly learned that a belief in maddening mothers failed to explain key facts about the illness. "Because of my sister," he said, "I had a firsthand contact with schizophrenia, and it looked no more like a psychosocial disease than diabetes does. The idea that it was psychosocial to me was absurd. What my sister had looked very much like a brain disease. It *was* a brain disease." In the 1960s and 1970s, as Torrey trained in medicine, he started looking at the epidemiology of the disease, and several things intrigued him.

As Torrey familiarized himself with the medical literature on schizophrenia, he was struck by cases of inpatients who had been admitted with diagnoses of schizophrenia but began limping a week or so after the beginning of their hospital stay, prompting staff to call in a neurologist. When the neurologist performed a lumbar puncture, the person turned out to have encephalitis, cytomegalovirus infection, or another infectious disorder. Acting on his insights, Torrey compiled cases that presented like schizophrenia or bipolar disorder but turned out to have a clear infectious basis, and in the 1990s he published a paper detailing them and their likely significance.

"To me, that was an important precedent," Torrey concluded. "While a medical student, I had learned that schizophrenia was seasonal, it was urban, and it looked like a lot of infectious neurologic disorders. It *looked* like an infectious disease."

Why, then, had not his more experienced professors grasped this? "Psychiatry is just like all parts of medicine; it has its fashions, and at that time the fashion was obviously Freudian or genetic," Torrey explained. "But it was one or the other, and if you wanted to be successful in your chosen profession, you knew you should follow what the senior people said. That was the way things were at that time.

"But"—he sighed—"how can I say this politely? I did not come out of my training with a strong belief that my senior colleagues necessarily knew what they were talking about. I think that's putting it as politely as I can."

But despite such insights, his attempts to reassure his mother that Rhoda's illness was not her fault were in vain. He was, after all, a recent medical-school graduate arguing against fervently held articles of psychiatric faith.

One could say that Torrey has sought to exonerate his mother and help his sister ever since. He decided to become a psychiatrist, and he chose schizophrenia as his focus. As his clinical experience mounted, he learned that schizophrenics suffer from puzzling physical deficits as well as mental symptoms; for instance, when a schizophrenic's gait was tested, she often staggered slightly and deviated from the straight and narrow, like a drinker over the limit. The presence of large numbers of lymphocytes, a type of white blood cell, indicated that their bodies were fighting inflammation. CT scans revealed enlarged ventricles in the brain, fluid-filled spaces within each hemisphere that expanded alarmingly as brain tissue was lost. But lost to what?

He received his psychiatric training during a period when Freud's psychoanalytic theories and Fromm-Reichmann's schizophrenogenic mothers were universally embraced, but Torrey pursued a very different vision of the illness that diverted his research attentions from psychology to infectious disease.[14]

As a psychiatrist, researcher, NIMH official, and, later, founding director of the private Stanley Medical Research Institute, Torrey has done more than spend his career unraveling the physical origins of schizophrenia. Probing, identifying, and documenting the infection at its core, he has also fostered a research climate that enables other investigators the world over to do the same; since 1989, SMRI has awarded more than $550 million in research grants to researchers in over thirty countries.

In 1980, a decade after Torrey's arrival in the Washington, DC, area, he partnered with infectious-disease expert and kindred spirit Robert Yolken, MD, of Johns Hopkins University. Among other research goals, the pair sought to discover which infectious agents could produce the physical deficits of schizophrenia. They considered Epstein-Barr virus, or EBV, which causes mononucleosis, nasopharyngeal carcinoma, and, rarely, Burkitt's lymphoma, an aggressive but curable cancer of the lymphatic system. Cytomegalovirus, or CMV, was another candidate, as it is easily passed from a pregnant woman to her unborn child, and so was *Toxoplasma gondii*, a unicellular parasite carried by house cats that is spread by undercooked foods and by cat litter and that at the time infected 20 percent of the people living in the United States. The duo also scrutinized influenza and herpes simplex virus type 2.

The schizophrenic subjects of Torrey and Yolken tended to harbor antibodies for these microbes, which provided evidence of an infection. But the researchers could find no actual microbes; the pathogens themselves eluded them, and they concluded that the infections must have occurred years earlier, leaving only antibody "footprints" to show the microbes had passed through.[15] Might infection have left its mark as early as childhood, infancy, or even in the womb? they wondered.

Back to the future

In their seemingly novel search for infectious causes of schizophrenia, Torrey and Yolken were in fact not crafting a new theory but updating an old, all-but-forgotten one.

How so? As chapter 1 disclosed, Sigmund Freud began his career as a neuroanatomist, but when he ceased scrutinizing brain structure to plumb the unconscious mind and develop the talking cure, he took the field of psychiatry with him.

Well, not *all* of it. For the first three decades after its discovery and labeling, schizophrenia, or *dementia praecox*, as it was then known, was regarded by many psychiatrists as a disease caused chiefly by infection.

The term *schizophrenia* was coined by Eugen Bleuler, a fin de siècle Swiss contemporary of influential psychiatrist Emil Kraepelin, who developed a categorization, or nosology, of psychiatric disorders in the late 1890s.[16]

Some turn-of-the-century doctors, including Kraepelin, associated schizophrenia with infection because psychosis was an occasional symptom of bacterial diseases like typhoid fever, tuberculosis, and diphtheria. In 1904, a review article observed that "insanity following infection is generally of short duration," but in some cases it was known to linger.[17]

Richard Noll, a clinical psychologist and historian of medicine, assures us that in the late nineteenth and early twentieth centuries, the dominant theories attributed schizophrenia to heredity and "intoxication," or poisoning, caused by focal infections of the sex glands, the intestines, and the mouth.[18]

Although Kraepelin's devotion to the infection model is often downplayed or ignored altogether, he might have been the theory's most famous proponent.[19] His 1895 text *Lehrbuch der Psychiatrie* speculated that dementia praecox was not a psychological issue but rather a "tangible" morbidity of the brain caused by autointoxication from pathological substances that were produced "somewhere in the body." It could be cured, he averred, by locating and removing the sources of this infection. Accordingly, Kraepelin recommended major abdominal surgeries,[20] such as the excision of (presumably infected) colons, as well as ovaries or testes and other organs associated with reproduction.

Although we identify Freud with the talking cure, even he indulged in a flirtation with surgery as a cure for psychiatric symptoms. As psychoanalyst Jeffrey Masson,[21] former director of the Freud archives, revealed, it proved disastrous. Having ascribed his Viennese patient Emma Eckstein's masturbation to a "nasal reflex neurosis," Freud and surgeon William Fliess performed a series of operations on the twenty-seven-year-old, removing portions of her nose to correct the putative nose malformation behind her sexual compulsion. Infections and other complications ensued, some due to errors such as failing to remove a gauze pack in her nose after surgery.[22] These complications nearly killed her and left her permanently disfigured "with the left side of her face caved in."[23]

Such gruesome outcomes did not quell psychiatrists' interest in the focal-infection theory. Two decades later, Chicago surgeon Bayard Taylor Holmes's research on schizophrenia led him to undertake corrective surgeries. In a once common, if ethically dubious, tradition,[24] in May of 1916, he performed abdominal surgery on his own child, his schizophrenic son, Ralph, twenty-six.

Four days later, Ralph died.

This did not stop Holmes, who continued to excise suspect organs and downplayed the tragedy of his son's death as he sought to popularize the surgical removal of organs to cure mental disease.[25]

In 1917, Holmes established the Psychiatric Research Laboratory of the Psychopathic Hospital at Cook County Hospital, where surgeries were performed on twenty-two patients with schizophrenia. Within ten months, two of them died.[26] Meanwhile, at Trenton State Hospital, Dr. Henry Cotton performed 645 major surgeries on patients with schizophrenia, manic-depression (bipolar disorder), and other psychiatric diseases. Thirty percent of them died—nearly one in three, a truly deplorable mortality rate.

The tragic deaths from surgeries meant to cure mental illnesses cast a pall over infection theories. Freud, who had distanced himself from such surgery after Emma Eckstein's mutilation, focused on developing a structural theory of mind, writing the *Interpretation of Dreams* and becoming the father of psychoanalysis. Infection theories were dismissed by his many acolytes, even after the discovery, detailed in chapter 1, that general paresis was caused by the syphilis bacterium.

But soon, a global crisis, the 1918–1920 influenza pandemic, made one infectious cause of psychosis impossible to ignore. The pandemic left in its wake a raft of psychoses and other mental disorders among survivors that dramatized the role of infection in madness. Influential Kansas psychiatrist Karl Menninger, who popularized psychiatry for the everyman, also declared his support for the infection theory.

Pandemic madness

The global influenza pandemic that began in 1918 supported theories that infection lay at the root of schizophrenia by providing dramatic evidence that infection—in this case, influenza infection—could result in psychosis.

The Spanish flu pandemic, as it was known, eclipsed the Black Death by killing fifty to a hundred million[27] people,[28] more than all the deaths in World War I. This dread global superbug began like a garden-variety flu, but within hours, the usual symptoms were compounded by dizziness, weakness, and pain.[29] The victim's inflamed mucous membranes and sneezing rapidly progressed to hemorrhaging, vomiting, and constipation.[30]

Cytokines, those signaling molecules that figure extensively in cellular communication, are known to respond to infection by recruiting immune cells to attack the invader, and some epidemiologists now speculate that the damage was due to an ill-fated cytokine storm as the bodies of the infected mounted a vigorous but ineffective assault against the virus.

Mental symptoms also abounded, according to frequent newspaper and physicians' reports as well as respected journals such as the *Journal of the American Medical Association*, or *JAMA*, which noted, "The frequency of mental disturbances accompanying the acute illness in the epidemic has been the subject of frequent comment."[31] As early as the 1890s,[32] the medical and popular conception of influenza had been changing to include a mental-illness component,[33] as physicians reported the "hypochondria, melancholia, mania, and depression that characterized general paralysis," or paresis. They also described anhedonia (a lack of enthusiasm for activities a person once enjoyed), loss of energy, apathy, and sadness.[34]

Moreover, a psychiatric symptom called nervous exhaustion, or *neurasthenia*, became the definitive symptom of influenza. Specialists[35] like London's Julius Althaus, senior physician at the Hospital for Epilepsy and Paralysis, began to compare influenza to paresis, opining that in both cases, the infectious agent attacked the nervous system to produce insanity.[36] Sir Benjamin Ward Richardson, a physician and the author of *Hygeia: A City of Health*, described influenza as an "epidemic neuroparesis" that generated "intense depression" in patients.[37] Even murders and suicides were attributed to the lingering legacy of influenza infection.[38]

The theory that infection might cause schizophrenia and other psychoses is bolstered by the fact that some of the 1918 flu survivors never recovered but instead developed a spectrum of lingering mental disorders, most notably postencephalitic Parkinson's syndrome.[39] Between 1915 and 1926,[40] an epidemic of *encephalitis lethargica,* also known as von Economo's encephalitis, attacked their brains, generating tremors, a slowing of physical and mental responses, profound personality changes, and even psychosis. Their psychiatric ailments included emotional disorders such as depression, anxiety, obsessive-compulsive disorder, and apathy.

These survivors of the 1918 flu pandemic sank irretrievably into psychosis and catatonia, and they were institutionalized, untreated, and forgotten as the century wore on.[41] "Interest in infectious theories of psychiatric disorders waned in the United States and Europe in the 1930s as Freudian theories became prominent,"[42] write Yolken and Torrey. Thus it was that fifty years after the pandemic, when Torrey proposed brain infection as a cause for schizophrenia in the 1970s, the precedent had been forgotten and the idea struck his psychiatric colleagues as absurd.

Undeterred, Torrey and Yolken compared normal and schizophrenic brains, probing them for evidence of inflammation and structural abnormalities (like enlarged ventricles), and, seeking the pathogens responsible, they focused on another signature of infection: seasonality.

A hibernal plague?

People born in the late winter and early spring, the peak flu season, are more likely than others to develop schizophrenia. The children born during cold-weather months in the Northern Hemisphere are also more likely to be exposed at an early age, either in utero or soon after birth, to microbes that are common during those months. This seasonal rise in schizophrenia risk is modest—only from 5 to 8 percent—but it has proven remarkably consistent across more than 250 studies. "How many psychosocial factors are going to give you a seasonality of birth?" asked Torrey. "The only seasonal birth patterns I knew were German measles, influenza, and other infectious agents, especially when the peak is in late winter and early spring: It just cried out 'infection!' The birth-month effect is one of the most clearly established facts about schizophrenia," continued Torrey. "It's difficult to explain by genes, and it's certainly difficult to explain by bad mothering."[43]

Thinking of cold-weather viruses puts people in mind of the flu, and indeed, influenza epidemics have been followed a generation later by waves of schizophrenia in England, Wales, Denmark, Finland, and other countries. The seasonal pattern also emerged when scientists studied people suffering from bipolar disorder, which is characterized by extreme mood swings, from euphoria to profound sadness, and seasonality emerged as a feature of multiple sclerosis as well. If these illnesses also turned out to be associated with an infectious disease that strikes in winter and early spring, the infection might explain the diseases' seasonality, wrote Torrey.

Torrey dedicated himself to identifying which pathogens triggered diseases like schizophrenia and bipolar disorder. He knew that fingering the microbial culprits was necessary if scientists were to prevent or even cure schizophrenia with a vaccine or a specialized antibiotic. Preventive strategies such as intensive prenatal care that stressed pathogen avoidance might also help protect future generations from schizophrenia. He knew that schizophrenia was a progressive disease and there was evidence that treatment mitigated its severity. Determined to unmask the offending viruses or bacteria, he embarked on what would be a decades-long microbial quest.

The laboratory advocate

Torrey cares about the fate of schizophrenics outside the laboratory as well. His research into schizophrenia's shrouded infectious origins is just one aspect of his zeal on behalf of the mentally ill. He became the prime catalyst in building the National Alliance for the Mentally Ill into a politically powerful advocacy organization, contributing the hundreds of thousands of dollars he earned from his successful 1983 handbook *Surviving Schizophrenia: A Family Manual.*[44] He has always given of himself, too, volunteering his services in the South Bronx, on a remote Alaskan island, and at Washington, DC, homeless clinics for several decades.

In his 1974 book *The Death of Psychiatry,* Torrey took his fellow psychiatrists to task for devoting themselves to the relatively minor concerns of the privileged "worried well," to the detriment of poor psychotics.

In his view, misguided policies such as deinstitutionalization, or "community psychiatry," which emptied mental institutions in the 1970s, contributed to homelessness, as it exacerbated the plight of the seriously ill, flooding the streets with people who were too sick to care for themselves. It's been suggested that "untreated psychiatric illnesses constitute one-third, or between 150,000 and 200,000 people, of the estimated 744,000 homeless population."[45] Torrey also denounced the profession for embracing theories that blamed devastated parents (like his mother) for their children's ailments. Families were grateful to Torrey, but this stance evoked bitter resentment from many members of his profession.

Torrey was careful to temper his criticisms with expressions of respect for his fellow practitioners, noting that, although Freudian models had not worked well, this negated neither the benevolence nor the good intentions of the healers who embraced them.

This was in contrast to the approach of his better-known contemporary Dr. Thomas Szasz, author of *The Myth of Mental Illness*. Szasz, who died in 2012, dismissed mental illness as a malicious invention of psychiatry that was used as an agent of control. A strong advocate for human freedom and individual liberty, he shocked the profession by arguing that mental illness was in no way a real disease akin to the physical disorders caused by bacteria or viruses. Szasz admitted the reality of only those few mental disorders with a clear biological pathology, like Alzheimer's. The others, he averred, were convenient fictions.

In his testimony to a U.S. Senate committee, Szasz not only decried psychiatry as an unalloyed agent of control but also compared doctors who incarcerated the mentally ill to prison wardens. "Since theocracy is the rule of God or its priests, and democracy rule of the people or of the majority, pharmacracy is therefore the rule of medicine or of doctors."[46]

Some lump Torrey in with Szasz, seeing in the latter's views a wholesale rejection of psychiatry and a *reductio ad absurdum* of

Torrey's theories. But in every important way, they are diametric opposites.

Torrey consistently expressed respect for both the reality of mental illness and the aims, if not the methods, of the profession. For him, mental illness was all too real, while Szasz denied the biological reality of schizophrenia and other serious mental diseases. Szasz's staunch defender Kentucky psychologist Robert A. Baker called Szasz "Psychiatry's Gentleman Abolitionist" in an article that dismissed the search for microbes that trigger schizophrenia, Torrey's holy grail, as "a category error analogous to attempting to photograph a dream."

For Szasz, the primacy of individual liberties led him to unilaterally oppose the forced treatment that Torrey regarded as essential to the health and recovery of many schizophrenics whose anosognosia caused them to reject the very medication they needed to remain well. Torrey definitively distanced himself from Szasz in the pages of the *New York Times,* calling him "a man who has produced more erudite nonsense on the subject of serious mental illness than any man alive."

Despite the more measured language with which Torrey criticized psychiatric theories and methods, his writings brought painful political consequences, forcing him to rely on his considerable resourcefulness. When the NIMH dismissed him in a political dispute over his writings, Torrey obtained the support of a wealthy couple whose son suffered from schizophrenia. With their funds, he established the Stanley Medical Research Institute, with himself as director and his patrons' son as its lawyer. He now commands a budget so massive that its disbursements rival the government's own, and he also controls the largest library of human brains in the world, which allows him to influence the direction of schizophrenia research by supporting selected researchers with these funds and neural tissues.

The enemy within

As Torrey and Yolken continued to ponder theories that might explain the seasonality of schizophrenia, French scientist Hervé Perron came into their orbit. Although still a doctoral candidate at France's Grenoble University, Perron jettisoned his PhD research topic when he became intrigued by the possible role of unusual agents called retroviruses in disease. Unlike DNA viruses, which take over cells by translating their DNA into RNA, retroviruses do the opposite, converting their RNA into DNA. Today, the term *retrovirus* is familiar largely because HIV is one, but in 1987, retroviruses were truly novel. So was Perron's theory that they were implicated in multiple sclerosis,[47] a disease that shows a seasonality similar to that of schizophrenia. Torrey and Yolken took interest.

Perron procured spinal fluid from many people with MS and tested it for reverse transcriptase, an enzyme used by all retroviruses. He found the enzyme and took electron-microscope photographs of the retrovirus that harbored it. Perron sought to identify the retrovirus.[48]

It was 1987 and the scientific world was catching up to Torrey. New research technologies, including neuroimaging, expanded the physical and metaphorical vision of scientists and helped to supplant the psychosocial view of schizophrenia with a focus on identifying distorted brain structures and function. Just as microscopes enabled sixteenth-century Dutch scientists to see various creatures that caused disease, powerful tools like magnetic resonance imaging, or MRI, machines visualize the brain with crystal clarity. Positron-emission tomography, or PET, scans showcase dynamic video images of the living brain. Scientists now agreed that they were looking at a brain disease.

Torrey and Yolken were in their second decade of seeking the microbes that cause schizophrenia, and Perron was still on a parallel track, seeking the retrovirus that seemed to be involved in multiple sclerosis. In 1996, eight years of sixteen-hour workdays paid off for Perron when he finally identified the responsible retrovirus. It was marvelous. Not only was Perron's discovery a previously unidentified viral factor in all MS, but it was also a previously unidentified *type* of virus. Unlike viruses that are normally borne on the breath, sneezes, blood, sweat, saliva, or semen of others, this virus is endogenous—it lives within us.

Because the virus Perron discovered lurks within the DNA of each of us, he called it human endogenous retrovirus W, or HERV-W. In the 1970s, scientists had been mystified to see viruses emerging from the cells of healthy baboon placentas in electron-microscope images.[49]

Unlike typical viruses, such as influenza, which kill the cells they infect, retroviruses allow the cells to live; they insinuate themselves inside, slipping their own genes into the cell's DNA so that future cell divisions will incorporate the retroviral genome. Perron estimates that perhaps sixty million years ago, a few million years after the dinosaurs disappeared, HERV-W slipped into the genome of one of our pre-simian ancestors, where it met with an uncommon piece of good luck: it landed in a germ-cell line that produced reproductive material—either sperm or eggs—and thereby assured itself of an entrée into all future generations; "a rare, random event," as Robert Belshaw, an evolutionary biologist at the University of Oxford, put it in *Discover* magazine.[50] Today, the human genome contains 100,000 of these viral squatters, which account for more than 40 percent of all human DNA.[51]

"Endogenous retroviruses are a very interesting set of agents," says Yolken. "To some extent, they're genes, part of the genome; to some extent they're viruses, because they're actually derived from viruses that infected our ancestors."

"This makes a disease they encourage *look* like a genetic disease," adds Torrey.

If HERV-W lives within us all, why doesn't everyone develop MS or the other diseases that endogenous retroviruses code for? Because our bodies are vigilant. We suppress endogenous retroviruses, preventing their translation into proteins and subsequent expression into disease by straitjacketing them, binding them tightly to coils of macromolecules. But occasionally a HERV-W virion escapes to crank out dangerous proteins and cause disease. When HERV-W does this, more than a dozen studies have shown, that person develops MS. Torrey and Yolken speculated that although our bodies normally restrain HERV-W, an infectious illness that strikes during the neonatal period can weaken the bonds that confine it.

As Perron triumphantly unveiled the mystery of MS and endogenous retroviruses, Torrey and Yolken considered whether retroviruses might also be culprits in some mental disorders. They knew by then that AIDS was caused by HIV, a retrovirus, so the duo investigated whether this retrovirus might trigger the psychosis experienced by many AIDS patients, who suffer symptoms that are also found in schizophrenia.

They found that the retrovirus they sought was HERV-W.[52] Several studies verified the presence of HERV-W in the brains and body fluids of people with HIV, and Perron's own follow-up study in 2008 revealed that 49 percent—nearly half—of people with schizophrenia harbor HERV-W, while only 4 percent of people without schizophrenia do.

Finally, after decades of searching, Torrey and Yolken had unimpugnable evidence that an infectious agent—the retrovirus HERV-W—played a key role in schizophrenia. This eureka moment was further heightened by the discovery that the retroviral concentration was proportional to the degree of brain injury, says Perron: "The more HERV-W they had, the more inflammation they had."[53]

A question remained: How does the same retrovirus produce MS and psychosis and raise the risk of schizophrenia, bipolar disorder, and severe depression? Torrey and Yolken theorized that the mechanism of the immune response, not the specific infectious agent, was key and that a number of pathogens might trigger schizophrenia. Accordingly, they determined to probe the roles of influenza, *Toxoplasma gondii,* and other microbes.

Poisoned wombs?

And yet, in a perverse manner of speaking, is Mother to blame after all? Do pathogens sow the seeds of schizophrenia in the womb, and if so, how? In one scenario outlined earlier, the fetus or newborn falls victim to friendly fire from its own immune-system defenses or from those of its mother. HERV-W may trigger not only schizophrenia but bipolar disorder and other illnesses.

Infection with herpes, toxoplasma, cytomegalovirus, influenza, and half a dozen other common pathogens release the HERV-W viruses, which flood the newborn's cerebral fluid and brain, ferrying proteins that can trigger an inflammatory response from the infant's fledgling immune system. White blood cells, which engulf or otherwise neutralize immune-system threats, emit cytokines, which are molecules that summon other immune-system cells in an attempt to vanquish dangerous intruders. But these immune cells can also attack healthy brain tissue, especially in infants and young children whose untutored or naive immune systems are less able to recognize and selectively assault invading threats.[54]

To test this theory, Perron injected HERV-W from people with MS into mice. The animals quickly lost their motor coordination, just as those humans with the disease do. After stumbling about for a while, the mice became paralyzed and then died of brain hemorrhages.

But if Perron first removed the immune cells known as T cells from the mice, they survived receiving HERV-W. This murine model illustrated an important variable: immune vigor. The immune system's purpose is to protect us from infectious threats by disabling pathogens. But in this case of friendly fire, the immune cells cause diseases, including schizophrenia, by attacking the person's own brain cells instead of the pathogenic invaders.

When Perron removed the animals' T cells, he prevented such injury, and so prevented the MS. This means that whether a person who is exposed to HERV-W will develop MS or schizophrenia may depend on his or her immune system's responses.

Like people with MS, people with schizophrenia seem to suffer profound but indirect damage from the inflammation created by their own immune systems. However, in schizophrenia, the neurons are overstimulated, not killed, which is why the symptoms of schizophrenia are more subtle. "The neuron is discharging neurotransmitters, being excited by these inflammatory signals," Perron explained. "This is when you develop hallucinations, delusions, paranoia, and hyper-suicidal tendencies."

In people diagnosed with schizophrenia, the cortical surface of the brain, the thalamus, the limbic system, and the basal ganglia shrink, while crevices called sulci and normally fluid-filled spaces, ventricles, enlarge by as much as 50 percent. Such changes may be the terrible legacy of a prenatal virus, although as Ian Lipkin, MD, director of the Center for Infection and Immunity at Columbia University, points out, people, including fetuses, may react very differently to infections. "A gunshot to the stomach is bad news for anyone, but microbial assaults yield more varied responses partly based on phenotype."[55] Factors such as genetic phenotype, age, general health, stress, inflammation, and the presence of environmental cofactors all affect an individual's susceptibility.

Crazy cats

"Schizophrenia was first seen in the late 1700s and first described clearly between 1808 and 1810 independently in both London and Paris. The bulk of people who described it said 'We haven't seen this kind of thing before,'" says Torrey. "I became completely convinced that schizophrenia was a relatively recent disease. I still am."

In his book *The Invisible Plague: The Rise of Mental Illness from 1750 to the Present*, Torrey reveals that around 1871, schizophrenia swiftly transformed from a rare to a relatively common disease. That same year, as U.S. schizophrenia rates rose sharply,[56] cat ownership became popular in England and America, as chapter 1 noted.

This is no coincidence, Torrey explains; cats transmit the one-celled parasite called *Toxoplasma gondii* to humans. *T. gondii* causes the disease toxoplasmosis, and it is already implicated in congenital illness when it infects a fetus.[57] Torrey and scientists on two continents think it does more; they think that a *T. gondii* infection causes schizophrenia.

In 1938, a newborn girl at New York City's Babies' Hospital became the first person to be definitively diagnosed with a *Toxoplasma gondii* infection, which she had acquired in her mother's womb. The parasite killed her within days, and doctors soon realized how dangerous *T. gondii* is for the unborn. It can not only kill outright but also cause children who are infected in the womb to be plagued by a congenital syndrome that includes deafness, retinal damage, seizures, mental retardation, and microcephaly (an abnormally small head).[58] They may also develop the disease toxoplasmosis, in which flu-like symptoms are followed by an inflammation of the brain, referred to as encephalitis, and various neurological deficits. Toxoplasmosis can harm the heart, liver, ears, and eyes as well. Because *T. gon-*

dii is transmitted by cats, obstetricians warn pregnant women who have cats not to touch litter boxes and to cook food thoroughly in order to kill any errant parasites.

Indoor cats can shed the parasite, so if they walk on surfaces that later hold food, the food can become contaminated. Playing with cats can lead to contamination if you don't wash your hands carefully before eating or placing your hands in your mouth. Outdoor cats that leave their feces on the ground also sometimes excrete into domestic animals' feed. This adulteration results in *T. gondii* tissue cysts within the animals' muscles. If humans eat this meat without cooking it thoroughly, they may become infected.[59]

So it is not surprising that one in every four U.S. residents is infected with *T. gondii*. In France the infection rate is about 50 percent,[60] thanks in large part to Gallic gustatory habits like a penchant for steak tartare and other forms of uncooked meat. In regions such as West Africa, the infection rate can soar as high as 80 percent.

Conventional wisdom long held that healthy adults who became infected weren't harmed, only those who were immunocompromised in some way due to HIV infection or some other illness. But Torrey and Yolken found that symptoms from headache to fever to anorexia were common even in adults with healthy immune systems.

Moreover, decades of human studies in countries such as the Czech Republic, Turkey, and Mexico have revealed that *T. gondii* dramatically changes the mental status of adults. Infected adults suffer behavioral changes that include increased recklessness, sexual attractiveness, sexual aggression, and receptivity. They also engage in risk-taking behavior that can be hazardous. For example, it makes the infected dangerous behind the wheel. In one Czech study, infected men were twice as likely as others to be involved in a traffic accident, while infected women seemed more than usually receptive to the opposite sex, a tendency that would certainly serve the parasite's purposes by increasing its spread to their sexual partners. A study of new mothers even revealed that infected women are more likely to commit suicide.

It's fortunate that we have human studies, because trying to evaluate subtle changes in cat behavior when they are infected with *T. gondii* reveals the limits of animal models, says Yolken. "How can you tell if a cat is crazy? Well, my daughter thinks that if a cat is nice and comes up to you when called and doesn't scratch the furniture, that would be a cat with schizophrenia.

"On the other hand we can ask questions about whether *T. gondii* changes behavior by looking at rat and mouse behavior: That can be done in animal models. Primates are more similar, so we might use chimpanzees or monkeys to investigate, but their changes are not the same ones we have, so we're limited in what we can do."

For decades, Torrey, Yolken, and their colleagues abroad, including Czech parasitologist Jaroslav Flegr, author of *Frozen Evolution: Or, That's Not the Way It Is, Mr. Darwin*, suspected that *T. gondii* caused subtle changes in an infected fetus that could lead to schizophrenia twenty years later. In 2008 Yolken and Torrey published a study indicating that the peak age for becoming infected by *T. gondii*, between eighteen and thirty-five, coincides with the peak age of the first signs of schizophrenia. They also noted that in areas where felines are rare, the prevalence rates of both toxoplasmosis and schizophrenia are low.[61] In 2005, studies in journals like the *American Journal of Psychiatry*[62] found that children of mothers who contracted *T. gondii* while pregnant did suffer higher rates of schizophrenia than other children. This is a highly suggestive association, especially because the parasite is known to be neurotropic—to target brain cells. Collectively, these studies strongly suggest that infection with toxoplasma is a significant risk factor for the development of schizophrenia.

So, fetal infection with *T. gondii* does correlate with higher schizophrenia rates. However, studies that followed people who moved from one region of the world to another found that their rates of both toxoplasma infection and schizophrenia reflected the rates in the part of the world where they'd spent their childhoods. In reviewing thirty other studies, researchers found that individuals who developed schizophrenia or bipolar disorder were significantly more likely to have grown up in a family that owned a cat, but not a dog, between that person's birth and age thirteen.[63]

Torrey found that the most strongly positive schizophrenia correlations were not with *T. gondii* infections acquired in the womb but with infections that struck children and teenagers.[64]

Why? What could possibly explain why childhood, not gestation or infancy, is when the young are most likely to acquire the toxoplasma that raises their risks of schizophrenia?

Torrey and Yolken blame sandboxes.

"A likely mechanism for exposure to *T. gondii* in childhood is playing in the dirt of sandboxes contaminated with *T. gondii* oocysts," they write, explaining that every uncovered public sandbox studied was used as a litter box by from four to twenty-four cats.[65] The cats shed *T. gondii* eggs and cysts that found their way onto the hands of children, who, being children, eventually put their unwashed hands into their mouths, ensuring *T. gondii*'s transit into their bodies.

The risk isn't limited to sandboxes, of course, because the same oocysts are found in the dirt and on outdoor surfaces on which children play. But the sandboxes provided convenient sites for research that showed how urban areas where cats had a high rate of infection became areas where later schizophrenia rates were similarly elevated.[66]

According to Flegr's studies, toxoplasma causes schizophrenia by affecting neurotransmitters in the brain, especially dopamine, glutamate, and GABA. For example, *T. gondii* increases the brain's dopamine levels by 34 percent, probably through the actions of cytokines, leading Flegr to describe dopamine as the "missing link between schizophrenia and toxoplasmosis."[67] The work of Flegr and others has implicated *T. gondii* in attention deficit disorder, hyperactivity disorder, and obsessive-compulsive disorder as well as schizophrenia.

The connection between toxoplasmosis and schizophrenia has positive implications for treatment because some of the antipsychotics used to treat schizophrenia are active against *T. gondii*. People whose schizophrenia is caused by *T. gondii* could be effectively treated by anti-infectives such as azithromycin, trimethoprim-sulfamethoxazole, and pyrimethamine-sulfadiazine.[68]

Torrey and Yolken think that both the influenza virus and *T. gondii* are likely triggers of schizophrenia and bipolar disorder. Perhaps they work via HERV-W as subsequent infections trigger the release of HERV-W, adding to the brain inflammation and causing schizophrenics to lose brain matter over time, as their enlarged ventricles—the spaces or "holes" in their brains—testify. "Enlarged ventricles mean that the brain is shrinking,"[69] declares a University of Toronto neurowiki site, and other parts of the schizophrenic's brain, including the thalamus and the insular cortex, shrink too.[70] If influenza and *T. gondii* infections trigger HERV-W release, this would explain why some schizophrenics are first diagnosed after an infectious illness[71] and why the disease, like MS, often waxes and wanes, with other infections causing an exacerbation of symptoms.

"Historically, rubella virus (which causes rubella, or German measles) would be on that list of agents that cause schizophrenia as well," says Yolken, but the vaccine has all but eliminated it in the West. Different agents cause psychoses, including schizophrenia, in different parts of the world. Malaria and rubella are likely culprits in the developing world, but Yolken also points out that "there are many infectious agents in the Third World that are unknown to us because studies have not been done."

"Typically, in animal models if you cure the toxoplasma, which we can do, the symptoms get better," says Yolken. "Preventing or treating *T. gondii* infection with a vaccine, on the other hand, is a great idea but it is a little further down the line."

Fetal infection

Children old enough to play in the pathogen-rich dirt are most vulnerable to acquiring mental disease, but earlier exposure— even before birth—can madden as well. The idea that the womb environment may exert lifelong effects on the fetus is certainly not new. In 1992, English epidemiologist D. J. Barker first argued that an undernourished fetus faces an increased adult risk of future heart disease. He also speculated that the same malnourishment somehow inculcates a tendency toward diabetes. Barker didn't offer much in the way of supporting data, but subsequent research has validated his observations, especially an analysis of pregnant women whose fetuses survived the famine of the Nazi-engineered[72] Dutch Hunger Winter of 1944–1945.[73]

A mother's high blood pressure, diabetes, and behaviors such as smoking and drinking are all implicated in fetal harm. Each may carry consequences, like mental retardation, diabetes, low or high birth weight, an increased heart-disease risk, or schizophrenia.[74] Of course, the father's medical conditions and behaviors may contribute heavily as well, but fewer studies have been done to document this.

In a joint study by Sweden's Malmo University Hospital and the National Institute of Mental Health, Thomas F. McNeil learned that trauma at the time of delivery, especially prolonged labor, appeared to affect an infant's brain structure, resulting in anomalies associated with schizophrenia.[75]

Infectious triggers do not exclude genetics as a risk factor, because genetics can be closely bound to immune response. For example, *Nature* published several studies implicating genes for human leukocyte antigens, or HLAs, in schizophrenia, positing that HLAs, not genes, control the production of neurotransmitters. Genes may also require a cofactor in order to be expressed, and a genetic response may determine who gets schizophrenia and who doesn't when an individual's immune system is presented with an assault by HERV-W.

Flu season

In the 1980s, Yolken and Torrey turned their attention to the common influenza virus. If neurasthenia was once accepted as a symptom of the flu and if the uncommon flu pandemic of 1918 resulted in psychosis, including schizophrenia-like symptoms, might the common flu trigger schizophrenia in infants and children?

Torrey has conducted carefully designed twin studies of his own to look for associations between influenza, schizophrenia, and bipolar disorder, and he also joined with Yolken to undertake several exhaustive reviews of decades of data[76] describing the offspring of women who had contracted influenza during flu epidemics. Dr. Alan S. Brown, a professor of psychiatry and epidemiology at Columbia, conducted large sophisticated analyses of blood assays from pregnant women who had actually contracted influenza, not simply those who'd been pregnant during epidemics.[77] This allowed him to more precisely associate infection with later schizophrenia among the offspring. A child whose mother contracts the flu in the first trimester of pregnancy, a period when the fetal immune system is relatively inactive, has a 700 percent higher risk of eventually developing schizophrenia; if the flu hits later, during the mother's third trimester, the child's risk of schizophrenia risk is "only" three times greater than that of the general population. Brown concluded that 14 percent of schizophrenia cases were the result of a woman's contracting the disease while pregnant. All these studies and more, Torrey says, tie schizophrenia to the common flu.[78]

Torrey hastens to note that not every researcher agrees with him, but he thinks it's most likely that only the mother is attacked by the virus, but her fetus falls prey to the antibodies she deploys against the infection. The antibodies secrete neurotoxic molecules that can damage the brain, and, in theory, the extent of this damage becomes apparent only as the brain fully develops years later and schizophrenia is diagnosed. In 2007, Paul Patterson and his colleagues at Caltech demonstrated the validity of this theory when they injected pregnant mice with a chemical that stimulated a strong immune response like that caused by influenza. It led to the birth of pups with behavioral symptoms associated with autism and schizophrenia.[79]

Yolken, however, issues a caveat: "I'm older, so as I always say, 'That's the $64,000 question. The big question.' We know they were infected, but we don't know *when* they were infected. So we can't know if the risk is only fetal infection or infection early in life."

Moreover, Torrey reminds us that the mechanism, rather than the specific infectious agent, determines the child's medical fate. The studies that implicate influenza in schizophrenia indicate that the virus plays a similar role in bipolar disorder and autism, and these studies have been replicated widely. Evidence strongly suggests that an assortment of biological villains, including herpes simplex virus type 2 (HSV-2), cytomegalovirus, and, perhaps, bornavirus, carried by horses in Europe, are all capable of causing the same slow devastation. Investigations of HSV-2 have yielded indeterminate findings, but Torrey and other researchers have widened their gaze to scrutinize rubella, which is already known to cause mental retardation and childhood psychoses.

Even in those cases where infection may be shown to cause mental disease, a role remains for genetics, stress, inflammation, trauma, and other risk factors that can render the brain more vulnerable to damage by infection. These actors combine in a synergy of risk to devastate the infected brain.

Germ theory as applied to mental illness is compatible with a role for genetics in schizophrenia, because genes may determine which brains are most vulnerable. Several infectious agents can cause the same disease, analogous to the situation where meningitis can be either bacterial or viral: Evolutionary biologist Paul Ewald suggests that we may one day speak of influenza schizophrenia or *T. gondii* schizophrenia and treat the disease accordingly.

Today, the evidence for a wide variety of pathogen-spread mental illnesses is copious and rigorous. That evidence is culled by advanced tools that Pasteur and Koch could only dream of. Functional MRI, or fMRI, allows dynamic imaging of the brain; antibody titers quantify infection indirectly by measuring the immune system's response to a pathogen; and high-throughput sequencing, an assortment of fast and cheap methods to sequence and analyze large genomes, enables the analysis of four hundred million base pairs of DNA in just ten hours.[80] Respected scholars at premier institutions have published clues to connections between various infections and autism, schizophrenia, obsessive-compulsive disorder, major depression, and more in peer-reviewed scientific journals. The evidence is mounting rapidly.

As bleak as this may sound, it's actually good news, because identifying which pathogens cause specific strains of mental illnesses will enable precise treatment. Determining the microbe's specific nature will allow researchers to target it with the most effective medication, just as discovering that HPV causes cervical cancer allowed scientists to devise a vaccine against this global killer. Antiviral medications and vaccines may quell influenza-induced schizophrenia, for example, while antibiotics can eliminate those cases of schizophrenia that are caused by bacteria.

Unfortunately, vulnerability doesn't end in early childhood. As the next chapter relates, adolescence brings its own array of infection-borne psychiatric disasters, from anorexia to OCD.

CHAPTER 3

Growing Pains: "Catching" Anorexia, Obsessive-Compulsive Disorder, and Tourette's

Moods and thoughts are just as biological as digestion and respiration.

— STEPHEN J. GENUIS

In March of 2013, I visited the offices of Susan Swedo, MD, in Building 10 of the sprawling Bethesda, Maryland, National Institutes of Health complex. This city of science houses everything from an army of investigators led by various public-health czars to support personnel to, of course, patients and subjects. I had always imagined this insular research kingdom as being nestled in some remote outpost, but the Washington, DC, Metro delivered me to its door.

After navigating the administration building's screening machines and humorless security guards requesting identification, I was photographed and permitted onto one of the shuttle buses that endlessly ply the NIH streets and parking lots. It reminded me of a border crossing.

Swedo graciously ushers me into the inner office of her Maryland clinic's suite. Although we've never met, we spoke in 1998 by telephone when I called to discuss her work for a *Psychology Today* article.

Then I had been struck by the forthright precision of her speech. Saved from severity by the faintest Midwestern twang, her hyperfluency was punctuated by gentle irony and sprinkled with easy laughter. Afterward, I looked for her image online out of curiosity—though I called it research—and was rewarded with a frisson of recognition: *Sissy Spacek,* I thought. *All-American girl.*

Sporting a chin-length reddish-blond bob, she looked directly at the camera through glasses, model-pretty but with a wide, guileless smile rather than the melancholic scowl of the fashionable. If her image has changed a bit over the decades, Swedo remains the perennial girl next door—if that girl were a medical prodigy who rose to become chief of the Pediatrics and Developmental Neuroscience Branch at NIMH.

Clad in a knee-length skirt and an impeccable white coat, Swedo, with her smilingly direct manner, appears conventional enough to play a doctor on television. Yet after speaking with me for a quarter hour in her office, she leans forward in her seat, looks directly at me, and crisply pronounces, "I'm not like most researchers."

As I'm sure my gelid smile conveys, I don't quite know what she means.

But over the course of the afternoon, a pattern emerges that sheds light on her claim. For one thing, I quickly discover that if you ask Swedo a question about herself, she'll end up telling you about a patient.

"How did you move from being a busy pediatrician who treated mostly underprivileged adolescents in Chicago mental-health clinics to heading a research wing at NIMH?" I ask, and in response she begins describing her odyssey from ambitious twenty-one-year-old medical student to newly minted MD juggling simultaneous positions in several Illinois adolescent mental-health clinics. But she quickly veers off into recalling the challenges faced by her first patients, including a sixteen-year-old from a well-to-do family whose fashionable mother couldn't be troubled to come to the hospital after her daughter's suicide attempt.[1]

When Swedo remembers this neglected child of thirty years ago, her eyes are bright with empathy, but what's audible is anger and impatience. "We are failing these children. How can you not *do* something?"

Instead of being festooned with the obligatory framed diplomas, testimonial letters, and conference posters that I've come to expect in doctors' offices, her walls are home to three mesmerizing thirty-by-forty-five-inch photographs taken by her husband, all images that glorify natural wonders. The sun-dappled florescence of lush, verdant woods enchants in one photo, while a nearly hyper-real shot that looks like Colorado's Pine Tree Arch radiates copper-hued glory and dominates a second wall. On the facing wall is a large frameless vertical triptych of angelically pretty, deeply saturated redheads—"my daughters." Atop a file cabinet against an adjacent wall, a seated persimmon-haired tot clad in an immaculate tennis sweater and shorts smiles into the camera, so beautiful and poised that at first I assumed that the image came with the frame. But this is her grandson. When I praise the red-haired beauties, she smiles broadly, then wistfully. "No one believes I was a redhead," she murmurs.

What really distinguishes Swedo's office, however, are the pandas. Two of the amply stuffed bears armed with hypodermic needles crown a massive bookcase; a grinning panda statue perches on a table edge exhorting well-child care; panda cartoons lampoon managed care; panda postcards litter a corkboard; and a panda poster announces a European conference on acquired mental illness after infections in adolescence.

It's fitting that pandas should dominate this otherwise lightly adorned space, because when Swedo is not speaking of her patients, she is speaking of PANDAS, which is, in a sense, another child that needs her protection and the key to helping her patients. To understand what PANDAS is, it's helpful to first hear the stories of some children who have been affected by it, like Seth.

A child's sea change

Flushed with irritation, Jane emerged from Seth's bedroom.[2] Until recently, her son had been a quiet ten-year-old whose small rebellions rarely went beyond balking at bedtime or objecting to limits on his Internet use. But this past week, life had become an endless series of complaints and arguments. Tonight he had refused to eat his dinner, complaining that the food "looked funny," and what if it were poisoned? He could *die*. First patiently, then angrily, Jane had sought to reassure him, and she finally gave up after a two-hour standoff during which he had resentfully pushed food around his plate without even pretending to eat it.

Now he wouldn't go to sleep. When she came in to turn off his light an hour after bedtime, this too became a tense debate. Seth had seen a documentary that included video images of rats running amok in the New York City subway and he whimpered that he was afraid of rats attacking him in the night.

Why was he behaving so childishly? she wondered. It was as if he were regressing, she thought, and she hated to admit it, but she was burned out on his nonstop whining and arguing. "There are *no* rats here. Go to sleep!" she snapped, turning out the light and slamming the door. As she headed down the hallway, she heard the light flick on again, and she stalked back, furious, and flung the door open.

"Rats don't like the light! They might not attack me if it's on. *Please* don't turn it off," Seth begged.

No more Discovery Channel for you, she thought wearily, and then, as the room came into focus, her heart sank. Seth was cowering on the far edge of his bed, his eyes continuously scanning the floor. She suddenly realized that behind his cranky recalcitrance and nonstop complaints, he was terrified.

She knelt by his bed. "Sweetheart, there's nothing to worry about. Would you like to sleep in my room; would you feel safer?" Nodding gratefully, Seth hugged her waist, and soon he was sleeping beside her. She too fell into a deep slumber, but later, she awoke to the empty depression where Seth had lain and to a strange, insistent sound. The clock read 5:15 a.m. As she padded out of the room, she realized that she was hearing running water and that she had been hearing it in her dreams for a long time, maybe all night. As the word *drown* flashed into her consciousness, she broke into a run.

But Seth stood before the sink, fiercely washing his raw, reddened hands in the running water with a worn shard of soap—it had been a new bar yesterday—a washcloth, and a coarse nailbrush. "Seth, honey, what are you doing?" she asked gently. "Please stop. Please." He didn't seem to hear her, and she knew what she had to do. "Come on, honey, you have to get dressed; we're going to the hospital."

When they arrived at the emergency department, she noticed that Seth's lower lip was twitching. He sat down but then leaped from his seat to pick up every piece of paper from the filthy floor with his raw, reddened hands, his head bobbing like a strange overgrown bird's.

Suddenly he stopped, transfixed, and then ran over and pulled her arm with all his might.

"Mommy, Mommy, they're coming to kill us! Let's go! Now! We have to go, now!" Jane tried to calm him, but she too was beginning to panic. Then the nurse called Seth's name.

Dr. Vogel, the pediatrician, told Jane that Seth had obsessive-compulsive disorder, or OCD. He explained that children with

OCD feel great anxiety and can't stop worrying. Repeating certain behaviors, like turning lights out in a certain order, tapping a certain number of times, or compulsively washing their hands, helps to allay their fears, and it's very difficult for them to stop these comforting rituals and behaviors.

Jane had heard of OCD, and she was relieved to have a name for Seth's bewildering behavior and learn that it was treatable. But she was also surprised that his symptoms had come on so quickly, virtually overnight. "Is this normal?" she asked Vogel, who responded that OCD was one of the most common childhood psychological disorders and a variety of things could trigger it, but Seth had probably had these inclinations for a long time; she had just been too close to him to notice the progression.

Jane didn't believe this. Seth had always been a placid child who smiled easily and who took skinned knees, reprimands, and playground frictions pretty much in stride. But this had changed recently, and the only unusual event in his life she could think of was several bouts with a sore throat. Seth had really suffered, spending whole days on the couch complaining bitterly about being sick, which was unlike him, unable to play, eat, or swallow without pain. As soon as one sore throat ended, another seemed to begin. After he'd been laid up with three, she learned that two of his classmates had recently recovered from strep throat. She belatedly realized that Seth, too, might have had this more serious strep infection, and she decided to take him to the doctor if he suffered another one, but he did not. He just became an anxious complainer.

Jane was racked with guilt to think that the two might be related: Would Seth have OCD now if she had taken him to the doctor for an antibiotic to halt his illness? But Dr. Vogel smiled indulgently at her fears and reassured her that Seth's problems were psychological. They had nothing whatever to do with a sore throat, strep or otherwise.

In 1994, when Seth was diagnosed, virtually all doctors would have agreed. Psychiatry recognized that children could fall prey to adult syndromes, from schizophrenia-type psychoses to anxiety disorders like OCD. Some psychiatric diseases, such as anorexia, affected children and adolescents disproportionately.

And in many ways, Seth fit the description of a typical child with OCD. The disorder typically strikes children around age ten, some of whom stop eating or fall into the grip of irrepressible tics, ceaselessly flexing their fingers, waving their hands, or jerking their heads arrhythmically while others, like Seth, begin to wash their hands over and over, even after the skin was cracked and bleeding.

Pediatricians ascribed diseases like OCD to psychosocial forces, and there was some evidence of a genetic predisposition; it ran in families. Even Tourette's syndrome, which plagues people with involuntary movements and utterances and is considered a genetic rather than a psychological disorder, is treated with talk therapy as well as antianxiety medication because it is so often accompanied by other psychological disorders.

Jane left the hospital with a prescription for an antianxiety drug and a suggestion that she take Seth to his pediatrician for follow-up.

Sitting in the pediatrician's Maryland office, Jane told the doctor that she just couldn't shake the idea of a connection between Seth's sore throat and the sea change. She knew her son, and this sudden transformation just felt, well, *biological*, to her; it felt like something that had happened to him, not something that he was. Or did every parent of an OCD child feel that way? She explained to the doctor that things had escalated very quickly: Seth had become more anxious as he recovered from these sore throats, suddenly developing nameless fears that kept him from eating or sleeping. Her messy son, Jane belatedly realized, had recently acquired a zeal for organization as well, categorizing and boxing his Legos instead of leaving them spilled across the floor of his room, alphabetizing his books on the shelf, and neatly hanging up the clothes that he'd once left strewn in piles. It hadn't occurred to Jane to regard this new-found neatness as a problem, but now, she thought of it as a symptom.

Jane half expected Seth's pediatrician to shrug off her worries as the ER doctor had done, but fortunately, Seth's pediatrician was Susan Swedo, who listened, intrigued, because Seth's story was unusual in ways that sounded familiar to her.

Swedo had been investigating Sydenham's chorea, a movement and emotional disorder that often arises after streptococci infections like a sore throat.[3] Sydenham's mostly affects children between ages five and fifteen. It is characterized by rapid, involuntary, spasmodic movements, mostly of the face, feet, and hands. The chorea, from the Greek word for "dance," refers to these movements, which are often accompanied by muscle weakness as well as emotional and behavioral problems. Seventeenth-century English physician Thomas Sydenham described the condition in the medical literature, but by then the disease already had a long history as St. Vitus's Dance, named after the patron saint of dancers. Our forebears knew of this illness as a compulsive *danse macabre* that they regarded as satanic in nature — it was a component of the devil's rites described during the Salem witch trials.

Sydenham's is now associated not with satanism but with rheumatic fever, or RF, which causes muscle aches, swollen and painful joints, a rash, and difficulty in concentration and writing. As many as 30 percent of children who contract RF develop Sydenham's, which, as Swedo knew, was the legacy of an untreated streptococcal infection. Although antibiotic use has rendered RF rare in developed countries like the United States, where it affects only one in every two hundred thousand children, it has recently made a comeback among the nation's undertreated, such as poor children in inner-city neighborhoods.[4]

Not only does Sydenham's follow streptococcal infections, but it is also seasonal, striking most frequently, like schizophrenia, during the winter and early spring. In the U.S., it is most common in the northern states.[5]

Swedo understood that the diagnosis of Sydenham's was fraught with opportunity for confusion, beginning with the specific nature of a child's involuntary movements, which are not simple tics and are not repetitive like the behavior of hyperactive children. They are truly random, small, contained "piano-playing" tics rather than the wilder gesticulations of children with other disorders. Also, Sydenham's is sometimes confused with cerebral palsy, which by definition is caused by some traumatic events during pregnancy or a baby's first year of life. By contrast, Sydenham's has a later onset, after an infection. Two clinical tests enable pediatricians to diagnose Sydenham's. In one, the doctor asks the child to stick out her tongue and keep it in that position; a Sydenham's patient will have trouble holding her mouth open and her tongue out for more than a second or two. In the other test, the doctor asks the child to squeeze her hand; a Sydenham's patient is unable to maintain a grip with steady pressure, so the child's hand will erratically tighten and relax, creating what doctors call the milking sign. Twice as many girls as boys are diagnosed with Sydenham's.

Because the rheumatic fever that results in Sydenham's is a rare complication of a strep infection, like the ones that Seth had weathered, Swedo wondered whether such infections were closely associated with other psychiatric symptoms — like Seth's OCD. She suspected that a syndrome might connect Group A streptococci, or GAS, infections that cause strep throat to a variety of childhood mental disorders.

She knew that for some children, psychiatric symptoms were the first harbingers of Sydenham's, as they became unusually restless, aggressive, or hyperemotional even before the physical symptoms of chorea, or dancing tic movements, appeared. Other symptoms were frequent mood changes, episodes of uncontrollable crying, behavioral regression—that is, acting like much younger children—mental confusion, general irritability, difficulty concentrating, and impulsive behavior. In the most common childhood psychiatric syndrome, OCD, intrusive thoughts, images, or impulses recurred, and children seemed powerless to abandon their compulsive behaviors. Often, affected children were seized by fears of harm coming to a family member or of intruders. They sometimes felt compelled to count silently, wash their hands over and over, organize items, or check repeatedly to ensure that a door was locked.

The rheumatic fever is itself a rare complication of a strep infection, and Swedo came to realize that such strep infections were closely associated with a repertoire of symptoms in OCD,

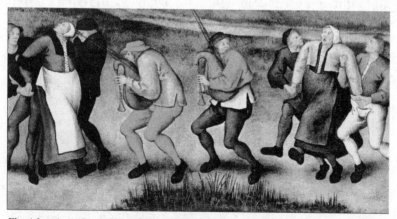

Flemish painter Pieter Brueghel the Younger (1564–1636) painted this representation of the dancing mania, also known as choreomania or St. Vitus's Dance, seizing a pilgrimage of epileptics en route to the church at Molenbeek. Such compulsive dancing was originally ascribed to satanic influence, and later to a collective hysterical disorder, but now seems due to infection of rye and other grains by the fungus Claviceps purpurea. *When people ate the tainted bread their symptoms included compulsive dancing. Streptoccocal infections also produced some cases.*

tics and Tourette's syndrome, anorexia, and other psychiatric illnesses. Were the GAS infections really triggering mental disorders? "It was like a mystery or detective novel," recalls Swedo. "I had to find out."

Swedo set about finding other children to whom this had happened and came up with a cache of children who had also suddenly become mentally ill, acquiring OCD symptoms or tic disorders shortly after a bout with strep throat or another GAS infection. As word spread that she was investigating the link, dozens of parents from the surrounding communities in the District of Columbia, Virginia, Maryland, and even as far away as Illinois and Michigan made pilgrimages to the NIMH complex to bring their anxious, OCD, anorexic, or tic-plagued children to her.

In 1995 Swedo's team at the National Institute of Mental Health studied a group of fifty children with OCD, both with and without tics. All their symptoms had been preceded by strep throat or a similar infection. When they tested these children, they found high levels of an antigen[6] (a substance that stimulates an immune response against a pathogen) that suggested a genetic susceptibility to rheumatic fever and to Sydenham's chorea.[7] Swedo found that these antigen levels were also high in children with autism.[8]

In 1998 Swedo published the landmark paper that laid out her theory of pediatric autoimmune neuropsychiatric disorders associated with streptococcal infections,[9] or PANDAS, that was afflicting normal children whose behavior exploded into madness within days, and sometimes overnight. First, they were paralyzed by an unfathomable anxiety. Without an apparent cause, this heart-stopping, unfocused fear of the sort that seized Seth was a harbinger of the full force of the psychiatric illness to come.

PANDAS is a syndrome, which means that it encompasses a number of disorders—OCD, Tourette's, anorexia, and others—

that share a cause. Swedo and other scientists estimate that PANDAS accounts for perhaps three of every twenty cases of such diseases. She cautioned researchers that PANDAS was not a default diagnosis and should be considered only in cases where the conventional model of illness did not explain a child's symptoms.

Such signs and symptoms include a rapid onset. In the case of PANDAS, symptoms arise a few days after infection; Sydenham's lag six to nine months behind. PANDAS symptoms show a gender disparity, with males more likely to have tics and females more likely to have obsessive-compulsive symptoms. Moreover, PANDAS children regress in ways that other Sydenham's, OCD, and Tourette's patients do not. PANDAS children suffer a rapid deterioration of fine motor control, as shown by loss of handwriting and drawing skills, whereas the decline is much more gradual in garden-variety, non-PANDAS-caused Sydenham's. A picture drawn by a sixteen-year-old PANDAS sufferer looks like the work of a six-year-old. This instant infantilism extends to other behaviors. Out of the blue, humiliated twelve- and thirteen-year-olds resume wetting the bed; some find that they cannot stem the flow of their urine even during the daytime. Preteens begin throwing tantrums, refusing to speak or eat, although the latter is often triggered by an unshakable conviction that their food is tainted or poisoned.

In 1998 I had felt excited as I read Swedo's PANDAS paper in the *American Journal of Psychiatry*; she had provided contemporary evidence for a broader role of infection in mental illness than I had imagined.

I already knew, at that time, that some mental disorders could be triggered by infection; the discovery—and rediscovery—that general paresis is one of the final devastations of syphilis is now common knowledge. Links between influenza and schizophrenia and between bornavirus and schizophrenia in Europe had also been discovered numerous times and just as consistently forgotten. I knew that contemporary psychoneuroimmunologists were wondering how much of the dementia and suicidal behavior in their HIV-infected patients could be attributed to the direct action of the virus on the nervous systems of the infected, rather than to the social pressures, despair, and medication side effects that were usually blamed. But in the late 1990s, human research into the microbial roots of madness seemed frustratingly sparse.

I wanted to know more, and Swedo was running studies in children, not petri dishes. She detailed how the body's response to an infection could go haywire in a young person with an inexperienced immune system, generating a vigorous but inaccurate friendly fire that damaged the body's own tissues instead of wiping out the invaders. In the model proposed by Swedo, antibodies that linger long enough interfere with functioning of the brain's basal ganglia.

How, I ask Swedo, did she gain this insight into the infectious nature of these childhood mental disorders? "It was a mom who first made the connection, not us!" she declared gleefully. "I always give her the credit because she, like other parents, know their children better than we ever can; if doctors will just *listen* to them, they can give us the answers."

The distinction between *patient* and *subject* is an ethically important one, but it is clear that Swedo's research subjects never cease to be patients in her eyes. The eagerness most researchers radiate when speaking of their theories is audible when Swedo speaks of the children and parents in her care and in her studies.

The fact that she puts her work as a pediatrician first has served her research well; Swedo pays careful attention to her charges, and her hypotheses grow from her experiences with them. Because some children with PANDAS suffered from tics after an infection—including grunts, vocal utterances, and even sometimes curses—Swedo began to think they might have a form of Tourette's as well.

About two hundred thousand Americans have the most severe form of Tourette's syndrome, or TS. It is named after Georges Gilles de la Tourette, the French neurologist who first described it in 1885. Usually diagnosed in children between three and nine years old, the neurological disorder is characterized by repetitive, stereotyped, involuntary movements and shouts, eye blinks, grunts, and curses or other vocalizations, even barking, that are collectively called simple tics. Some experience more complex motor tics that include facial grimacing combined with a head twist and a shoulder shrug. Tics are often worse during periods of excitement or anxiety and better during calm, focused activities. For such a rare disorder, TS has received a surfeit of media attention since the 1970s, and as many as one in every one hundred U.S. residents now report milder symptoms of TS such as tics, or involuntary sudden, brief, repetitive movements that involve a limited number of muscle groups.

There are no blood, laboratory, or imaging tests for a TS diagnosis. Instead, children are diagnosed when they have suffered both motor and vocal tics for at least one year. TS is chronic in 10 to 15 percent of affected people but most children who are diagnosed exhibit the worst symptoms in their early teens, and the tics gradually subside as they enter adulthood.[10] This provided solid evidence of a connection to PANDAS in Swedo's eyes, but more studies were necessary to prove the causal relationship and to characterize the mechanism by which GAS caused mental disease. Importantly, Swedo sought to discover whether treatments for GAS infections, such as filtering antibodies from the children's blood, would reliably alleviate the children's PANDAS symptoms.

As she recruited more children who had had experiences like Seth's, the word spread through pediatricians' offices, support groups, and mommy blogs, the theory resonating with many parents who felt that insidious infections, not genetics or family tensions, were behind their children's OCD, anorexia, or Tourette's.

On one such blog, a mother from Flint, Michigan,[11] shared the story of her daughter's sojourn in OCD hell.

One July day, Bertha, her "outgoing, friendly, and spunky" nine-year-old daughter, "woke up transformed" into a toddler, erupting in screams, tantrums, and whining at the slightest frustration. Bertha reverted to bed-wetting and baby talk and seemed tortured by a compulsion to repeatedly touch surfaces and door handles, crying, "Mommy, Mommy, help me, I can't stop doing this!" Even her handwriting and drawing reverted to that of a three-year-old.

"It was as though she was possessed," wrote Bertha's mother. Her daughter was diagnosed with OCD at ten years old, the typical age of onset.

But Bertha's overnight descent into illness seemed unnatural, and her mother was convinced that something physiologic was afoot. While Bertha took medication and saw a behavioral therapist, her mother read everything she could on the subject, and one day she stumbled upon the PANDAS theory and Swedo's NIMH studies. She drove her daughter to Maryland, where Bertha joined a study of twenty-seven children with obsessive-compulsive disorder. The treatment involved filtering the offending antibodies from the children's blood. Swedo used immunomodulatory interventions, including steroids, intravenous immunoglobulins, and plasma exchange, to treat the underlying infections in carefully controlled clinical trials.

Like most of the study's subjects', Bertha's symptoms abated. Almost immediately she was able to resist the compulsions, and as her antibody levels fell, her verbal expression and drawings drew near the age-appropriate level. Within a month, her normal speech and bubbly demeanor resurfaced, and she was restored to her family. Of the eighteen children diagnosed with PANDAS who were treated similarly, all but two improved. Seth, whose mother had first glimpsed the connection between his sore throat and a mental disorder, was among them.

This improvement is important because it helps bridge the gap between correlation and causation. Not only are the high antibodies to the infection associated with the mental-illness symptoms, but as the antibodies are banished, the symptoms abate, which suggests a causal relationship between the madness and the antibodies and, therefore, between the madness and the infection.

A mania for thinness

Another PANDA illness that strikes mostly girls is the queen of childhood psychological disorders.

Ten-year-old Greta sprang out of bed, grateful for the flood of early-morning sunshine through her window. The cold climate and usually gray skies of Rochester, New York, rarely gave way to such glorious weather, even in mid-May. She swallowed tentatively, then smiled; her throat still felt completely better. April had been cold and rainy, and she'd kept getting sore throats, one after another. Until a few days ago, she'd also had sharp stomach pains that came and went without warning. Luckily, they'd faded just as her mom began speaking of taking her to the doctor. At least her appetite hadn't returned, a good thing, because Greta was seriously dieting. She was determined to be a size 6 by September, when she would turn eleven. Lately, she could think of nothing else.

Donning her plaid shorts, the "lucky pants" she'd taken to wearing every day, she was gratified to see how loose they were.

She drank her daily cup of nonfat milk, or half of it, and quickly jumped on her bike to burn it off. She soared through the streets of her small city, going past the university, and eventually reached the village green of a suburb nine miles away. Slowly wheeling her bike down Grand Street to rest, she peered into the windows of the upscale boutiques and dreamed of the day she would be able to wear such clothes. But first she had to lose weight. The thought made her stomach clench for a minute, but then she remembered how loose her shorts were; she was on her way.

Suddenly she longed to weigh herself, so she pedaled home as fast as she could, drank the rest of her milk, iced, and called it lunch. Only then did she allow herself to get on the scale — she saw she'd lost a pound since yesterday. She frowned; not enough. She'd skip the cup of spinach she'd taken to eating for dinner every day and go for another ride in an hour or so. Greta then began her regimen of daily sit-ups.

By September, Greta was a size 4! On her relatively tall five-six frame, this looked thin, but she didn't think so; compared to the models in magazines, she was still too fat. She did think she looked like a different person, though, and she felt all eyes on her. When a few people, including her favorite teacher, took her aside to warn her not to lose too much weight, she wanted to laugh; she still had far to go. She'd set her sights on becoming a size 2 before Christmas. Every time she thought of her new goal, she rapped twice, softly, on her desk; somehow, this helped reassure her that she would achieve it.

Greta didn't know it, but she suffered from anorexia nervosa, often referred to as simply anorexia or AN. She was so obsessed with weight control that she ate only very small quantities of certain foods, which resulted in an abnormally low body weight. Like other eating disorders, anorexia is a disease of young people; 95 percent of those who develop eating disorders are between the ages of twelve and twenty-six,[12] and anorexia is the third most common chronic illness among adolescents.

The anorectic's distorted body image makes her see herself as overweight no matter how thin she becomes. Her relentless pursuit of thinness is accompanied by obsessive thoughts about food, calories, and weight. To allay this obsession she frequently engages in self-weighing, compulsive exercise, or even binge eating followed by extreme methods of purging the food, such as vomiting, enemas, or laxatives. Unusual eating behaviors, such as eating only raw green vegetables or only even numbers of grapes, are common.

Although some with anorexia nervosa recover after one treatment session, others go on to develop chronic illness. Their health declines, their menstrual periods stop, their hair and nails become dry and brittle, and their internal body temperature drops, causing them to constantly feel cold. These symptoms are followed by weakness, anemia, muscle wasting, and low blood pressure, and finally the victim suffers heart, brain, and other organ damage, which can be irreversible and result in death.

OCD and anorexia are related not only by their compulsive symptoms but also by the way neurotransmitters malfunction in both.[13] What's more, as in OCD and Tourette's, some cases of childhood anorexia are triggered or dramatically worsened by GAS infection, placing this autoimmune species of anorexia under the PANDAS umbrella of disorders.[14]

Anorexia is usually treated by medical monitoring and nutritional counseling with individualized psychotherapy, including cognitive and behavioral approaches that are tailored to the disease. The FDA has also approved antidepressant medications as part of the treatment.

Anorectics can be completely cured,[15] yet in 2009 the *American Journal of Psychiatry* reported that one of every twenty-five people treated for anorexia nervosa dies of the disease,[16] and the number of deaths due to anorexia may be even higher, because relatively few sufferers are formally diagnosed.[17]

As many as 90 percent of U.S. anorectics are girls, and male anorectics are far less likely to seek treatment because of the perception that it is a woman's disease. Because eating disorders have the highest mortality rate of any mental illness,[18] we need more and better treatments for anorexia. Researchers have discovered that anorexia is caused by a complicated mixture in which genetics, psychology, and social factors interact. But GAS infection may be an underacknowledged biological risk factor for anorexia, and addressing it might save people who are not helped by psychotherapies.

Brain imaging and genetic studies may provide clues to how each person develops the disorder. Such knowledge may allow researchers to create specific treatments for preventing and curing infection-driven medical anorexia.[19] For this to work, doctors would need a means of identifying the PANDAS anorectics.

In 2000 Swedo reported in the *Journal of Child and Adolescent Psychopharmacology* that she'd tested four children who showed the clinical signs of having PANDAS anorexia and found the same antigens that were elevated in the other PANDAS disorders, indicating the telltale GAS infections.[20]

Mistaken identity?

PANDAS doesn't cause every case of OCD, or even most of them. In fact, current research ascribes just one in ten cases of OCD and Tourette's to PANDAS.[21]

Or maybe, some critics scoff, no cases at all. Swedo's article was met by an initial acceptance and a flurry of corroborative studies. Most of the 173 articles focusing on human PANDAS studies I found on PubMed cite researchers convinced that

PANDAS is real—convinced enough that they continue to refine, quantify, and augment the diagnosis and mechanism.

But some scientists were skeptical from the first, and soon enough the PANDAS theory was roundly assailed. Some questioned whether the connection was really causal, noting that the frequent sore throats characteristic of PANDAS cases are too common to constitute a distinguishing feature of the syndrome, especially because some children are never diagnosed with strep throat.

Perhaps, the naysayers suggested, Swedo was confusing garden-variety movement disorders—such as Sydenham's and Tourette's—with the PANDAS movement disorders. Might they not be the same disease?

This question seems illogical because it ignores Swedo's admonition, even in her earliest PANDAS writings, that doctors must first rule out the normal varieties of these illnesses before deciding that a child may have PANDAS.

And she scoffs at the suggestion that she has confused common movement and psychiatric disorders with PANDAS when in fact she has painstakingly tracked the differences.

For example, the onset of typical OCD is gradual, even insidious, taking months or years to manifest, while the dramatic OCD symptoms of PANDAS spring up literally overnight. PANDAS is frequently preceded by an incapacitating fear and anxiety that persists through the illness. Parents often report that a child can remain relatively symptom-free at school, only to explode in a fit of anxiety and aggression when he arrives home, immediately consumed by frightening rituals and tics. Typical OCD strikes children around age ten, but PANDAS sufferers can be half that age. And in Tourette's and Sydenham's, Swedo says, "the movements are *very* different. The choreoatheoid movements of Sydenham's chorea are random, purposeless, snake-like writhing movements or quick muscle jerks and jumps that interrupt a volitional movement,[22] while the choreiform movements that characterize PANDAS are small 'piano-playing' movements of the fingers that are seen only in certain postures."[23]

The theory that GAS causes many of the intractable mental disorders of adolescence—OCD, Tourette's, anorexia, autism, and others—has suffered a backlash that has forced Swedo and others who treat and research PANDAS to address questions about study design, the suitability of animal models, and the very nature of proof.

"Several excuses are always less convincing than one," noted Aldous Huxley, and some critics ask how GAS can cause so many different mental disorders. Might it not be more logical to regard these very common bacteria not as causative agents but loiterers at the scene of a crime committed by some more conventional trigger of madness—stress, trauma, or genetics?

The belief that PANDAS needlessly complicates the diagnoses of garden-variety anorexia and Tourette's invokes Occam's razor, a scientific concept stating that even far-fetched theories are unnecessary when a simple explanation will do. As thirteenth-century philosopher William of Occam insisted, when theories compete, the simplest is preferred. The medical shorthand is "If you hear hoofbeats in Central Park, don't think of zebras."

The versatility shown by PANDAS, however, implies a survival strategy that should not be surprising in pathogens. Microbes, more rapidly driven by evolution than humans, display an impressive adaptive range of effects on their hosts, but their hosts are players in the evolutionary game too, so not all strategies end up improving the microbes' lot. Strains of the human papillomavirus, or HPV, promote warts and cancer of the cervix, penis, and anus, as well as cancers of the head and neck. Epstein-Barr virus causes mononucleosis, Burkitt's lymphoma, and Hodgkin's disease. *Helicobacter pylori* causes both ulcers and heart attacks when it is not protecting against obesity; *Clostridium botulinum* brings on rapid death by paralysis, but it also seems to alleviate depression, as noted in chapter 6; *Porphyromonas gingivalis* causes heart disease and gingivitis; *Chlamydophila pneumoniae* triggers heart disease and pneumonia; and *Streptococcus mutans* causes not only dental decay but heart disease.[24]

Moreover, PANDAS relies not on a direct infection but on collateral damage; the maladaptive *response* to infection can trigger different neurological effects depending on which structures of the basal ganglia it harms.

These ganglia are interconnected areas of the forebrain that cooperate to control voluntary movement, learning, some habits, emotions, and thinking. The basal ganglia control motor neurons that generate movement and are also thought to control action selection, or *intentional* actions. When these ganglia are hampered in moderating the body's motor systems, the person is racked by involuntary uncoordinated motions.[25]

Biological... and benign?

As I read the blogs, support-group posts, and online personal videos by parents struggling with their children's sudden, mysterious symptoms—and even by children who suspected that they might have PANDAS—I was astonished to discover how many wrote of hoping that they would be diagnosed with the syndrome, which would neatly explain their woes and present a course of action. Many, in fact, wrote of feeling dismissed after receiving other diagnoses, such as mass hysteria or malingering. Even worse, some received no diagnosis at all, just a baffled therapeutic silence. An actual diagnosis with a tangible cause—PANDAS—was, for many of these families, devoutly to be wished.

It's easy to understand why people are eager to identify their illnesses with PANDAS. For many, a biological cause is far easier to sympathize with than a mental-illness diagnosis, which still carries a stigma for not only the sufferer but his or her entire family.

In biblical times, people asked as a matter of course what sins had been committed by the mentally ill person or his parents to explain his symptoms, and as I've noted, Sydenham's chorea was known as a satanic *danse macabre*. Now we know that in many cases it is the fruit of a Group A beta-hemolytic streptococcus infection.

But a stubborn moral taint lingers. As chapter 2 explains, as late as the 1980s, psychosis was still being blamed on "schizophrenogenic mothers," and autism was still being ascribed to poor parenting; *someone* had to be to blame. By contrast, mental disorders with a biological basis, such as influenza, bornavirus, and GAS infection, seem morally neutral. Children get infections as a matter of course; no one blames the parents or accuses the victims of intellectual or moral weakness.

"When I practiced medicine at Children's Memorial Hospital in Chicago, I saw parents suffer horribly when they lost their children to leukemia," Swedo recalled. "When I came to the NIMH, I began to see parents lose their children to OCD and schizophrenia. These parents' grief is so much more profound. The fact that their children's illnesses are socially unacceptable makes their pain almost unbearable."[26]

The desire for the morally neutral refuge of a biological cause may explain why people with symptoms who identify themselves as having PANDAS but who do not meet the criteria express impatience or frustration with doctors. Parents often insist that doctors miss the diagnosis because they are unaware of PANDAS, not because the ill person does not meet the diagnostic criteria. And when children with symptoms of OCD, anorexia, Tourette's, or anxiety do not meet the criteria for PANDAS, they and their parents often resist hearing this, perhaps because a PANDAS diagnosis can represent an escape for the whole family from the stigmatized label of *mentally ill*.

In short, people with PANDAS have begun to claim new identities as victims of a biomedical brain disease as that explanation for their madness gains greater sympathy from the public.

PANDAS offers an alternative identity in the manner described by philosopher Ian Hacking, who has written of how new labels of mental disorders are embraced as redefinitions that allow people to escape the confines of labeling or loosen the shackles of stigma.[27]

There are precedents. In 1968, for example, around the time that the *Diagnostic and Statistical Manual of Mental Disorders* deemed homosexuality a mental disease, the creation of the homosexual as a specific kind of person was often traced to a paper by Mary MacIntosh entitled "The Homosexual Role,"[28] published in *Social Problems,* a journal that Hacking says "was much devoted to 'labeling theory.'" Hacking's article asserts that social reality is "conditioned, stabilized, or even created by the labels we apply to people, actions, and communities."[29] Similarly, multiple personality disorder, describing a syndrome in which a person is plagued with several identities, was invented around 1875, after which people flocked to become diagnosed with the disorder. Theories abound as to why people sought out the diagnosis, and the motivations probably differ from person to person. But people often find a diagnosis, almost any diagnosis, more comforting than grappling with bewildering mental symptoms that make them fear for their sanity. The role of clinicians is also important because psychiatry has its trends and fads, leading many symptom-ridden patients to receive whatever diagnoses are currently in fashion.

As we've seen from the stubborn bias against homosexuals and their former characterization as "mentally diseased," a redefinition does not always banish stigma or mistreatment. Recasting mental illness as a form of infection can also backfire, especially in the case of especially dreaded or sexually transmitted diseases. When syphilis was demonstrated to cause paresis, judgment rained down on paretics, and the STD stigma may even explain the willingness of researchers of the time to engage in malaria therapy, infecting paresis sufferers with a chronic and debilitating disease. Tuberculosis, by contrast, was morally rehabilitated after it was discovered to be infectious. Before that, TB was referred to as consumption, which, says Hacking, "was not only a sickness but also a moral failing, caused by defects of character. That is an important nineteenth-century social fact about TB. We discovered in due course, however, that the disease is transmitted by bacilli that divide very slowly and that we can kill." The idea of the consumptive as "a particular kind of person" with certain character traits, rather than simply a person suffering from illness, was, Hacking says, "an artifact of the nineteenth century."[30]

But several studies have determined that, even when the infections themselves carry no social taint, "emphasizing the biological aspects of mental illness does not reduce stigma and discrimination among the general public."[31] Although ascribing mental disorders to frankly physical causes like brain-chemistry imbalance or infection is an approach that discourages the assigning of blame for illness, this also promotes the belief that the illness, being biological, is intractable. As an article in *Schizophrenia Bulletin* explains, such biological underpinnings foster the belief that the sick person is impervious to treatment and therefore may be dangerous.[32]

Medical professionals harbor their own brand of prejudice, and their discrimination against mental disease is a product of the very mind-body dualism that has prevented the profession from recognizing the infectious contributions to mental illnesses in the first place. Toronto mental-health commissioners Thomas Unger and Stephanie Knaack explain why:

When presented with a symptom or set of symptoms, for example, physicians will start by using the fundamental schematic categorisation of "Is it functional or is it organic?" If categorised as organic (i.e. in the body) it is assumed to be real, legitimate and material. From the physician's point of view, this means it is something that can be observed, studied, treated and corrected. Arguably, this reduces stigma and discrimination. However, if categorised as functional (i.e. a problem of the mind, with no physiological correlates), the physician will consider it less real and the patient may be more likely to be stigmatised and discriminated against.[33]

For those with mental diseases caused by infection, better treatment may be in the offing, because the infection and its damage present a discrete medical target, unlike the murky but widespread theories of brain-chemistry imbalance that have not always held up well to researcher scrutiny.

A contested diagnosis

Sydenham's is known to be caused by childhood infection with Group A beta-hemolytic streptococcus, and it affects 30 percent of children who suffer acute rheumatic fever. But unlike Sydenham's, causation in PANDAS remains contested.

It's not that anyone questions whether the affected children were infected with GAS; Swedo and others have rigorously documented the presence of antibodies to the bacteria, although less sensitive tests by doctors who are not PANDAS specialists may fail to detect them. Skeptics, however, attack every other tenet of the theory.

They ask, "Is PANDAS really distinct from garden-variety Tourette's and OCD?" and point out that the discovery of

PANDAS was made from case-finding among sick children who fit the general profile rather than from forward-looking studies of large numbers of children gathered at random, and some wonder whether this method creates an illusion of causality.

The ubiquity of GAS also works against the PANDAS theory in the eyes of some. One can see for oneself that strep throat and related infections are everywhere but Tourette's and OCD are not. Does this mean that GAS infection is a cofactor, insufficient to cause disease on its own but exacerbating the damage from genetics, stress, trauma, or even poor parenting? Or is GAS just a near-ubiquitous innocent bystander? To those convinced of PANDAS's disease status, it is clear that not everyone with GAS becomes mentally ill because many factors affect vulnerability. Genetics, immunological vigor, general state of health, and perhaps environmental insults may all determine who develops PANDAS and who is able to avoid antibody damage to the basal ganglia.

Correlation and cause are two different things; for strep infections and PANDAS, the former has been demonstrated, but the latter is proving far more elusive. Correlation is the Achilles' heel of research into disease causation. Heart disease, for example, is strongly associated with stress. But do people suffer from heart disease because they are stressed, or are they stressed because they suffer from heart disease? Or is there some more complicated explanation for why stress and heart disease are frequent traveling partners?

Here is one example of the difficulty of teasing cause from correlation: Studies done before 1992 revealed that hypochondriacs were much less likely than their peers to develop atherosclerosis, or hardening of the arteries. Leaping to a narrow causative explanation, you may conclude that excessive worrying about your health is good for your heart. But in 1999, a *Jour-*

nal of the American Medical Association study showed that tetracycline use is associated with a lower incidence of heart attacks.[34] People open to broader analyses may reason that because hypochondriacs are more likely than others to take antibiotics to ward off infections, and because the atherosclerosis associated with heart disease is caused by various bacteria, it may be the antibiotic, not the worrying, that is protective. And they're right. Hypochondriacs are less likely to develop atherosclerosis because they are more likely to take the antibiotics that knock out heart pathogens such as *Porphyromonas gingivalis* and *Chlamydophila pneumoniae*.[35]

A lack of consensus

Swedo seems dismayed by the vigor with which critics like Harvey Singer, the Haller Professor of Pediatric Neurology and director of Child Neurology at Johns Hopkins, chip away at PANDAS. How do you prove an infection causes an illness?

"We need consensus," she explains as we sit together in her office, "and we had a meeting at NIH in July 2010 to reach agreement on the clinical picture of the acute-onset cases. Unfortunately," she snaps, tapping a paper impatiently, "three of the forty-one attendees elected to publish a 'minority report' entitled 'Moving from PANDAS to CANS' (childhood, rather than pediatric, acute-onset neuropsychiatric syndrome) and the debates intensified, rather than being resolved by the meeting."

This is yet another paper criticizing the evidence behind the PANDAS model and proposing an utterly different model and acronym, CANS, that removes any reference to an infectious agent.[36] Swedo has circled all the paper's points that, in her opinion, do not accurately reflect the evidence; coarse black circling fills the pages.

But compelling evidence must accompany consensus, and attaining traditional proof is hampered by research constraints. Ethically, you can't infect people with GAS and wait for symptoms to develop. You can't remove people from every other known risk factor for insanity—genetics, stress, inflammation, brain damage—to see whether GAS alone triggers it. The usual methods of proving medical theories seem infeasible.[37]

Further questioning PANDAS's disease status, some pointedly note that neither PANDAS nor its newest incarnation, the very similar pediatric acute-onset neuropsychiatric syndrome, or PANS,[38] is a disease entry in either the International Statistical Classification of Diseases and Related Health Problems (ICD) or the psychiatrist's bible, the *Diagnostic and Statistical Manual of Mental Disorders*.[39] The current edition, the *DSM-5*, defines a mental disorder only as "a clinically significant behavioral or psychological syndrome or pattern that occurs in an individual [which] is associated with present distress...or disability...or with a significant increased risk of suffering." In the case of PANDAS, the *DSM-5* refused to commit itself, noting that it remains a controversial diagnosis, citing both the PANS (Swedo's) and CANS (Singer's) revisions to the clinical picture.

Straddling the fence

But this failure to endorse PANDAS/PANS means little, because the wheels of psychiatric epidemiology turn glacially slowly. The *DSM* in particular is quite malleable and tends to reflect the sociopolitical climate as much as the medical one, so a disorder's inclusion or banishment from the manual follows closely on the heels of its political fortunes.

Witness the removal of homosexuality as a mental illness, which took place only after gay-rights activists demonstrated at the 1970 American Psychiatric Association meeting in San Francisco. By 1973, *homosexuality* was removed and replaced by *sexual orientation disturbance.*

Today a political furor swirls about the *DSM-5*'s consolidation of autism, Asperger's syndrome, and similar conditions within the overarching category of autism spectrum disorder, or ASD, which affects one in eighty-eight U.S. children. "The change signals how symptoms of these disorders represent a continuum from mild to severe, rather than being distinct disorders,"[40] notes APA literature, but its new definitions also reduce the number of people who are diagnosed with autism-like ailments such as Asperger's syndrome by nearly one-third, according to a Columbia University study in the *Journal of Autism and Developmental Disorders.*[41] There's much dissension from those who fear this "may leave thousands of developmentally delayed children each year without the ASD diagnosis they need to qualify for social services, medical benefits and educational support," as the Columbia researchers predict, and although the *DSM* editors wrote that this consideration did not figure in their decisions, they had to be aware of it. The change is also problematic for adults who identify with their Asperger's diagnosis. They stand to lose not only material resources and employment protections but the psychological and social benefits of a diagnosis that runs social interference for them. An awkward or standoffish person with a diagnosis of Asperger's is likely to be met with more respect and understanding than someone who exhibits the same behavior but is unprotected by a diagnosis; people may think he is simply unfriendly or judgmental.

The *DSM* has its medical flaws as well, according to critics who decry its invalid and inconsistent "cookbook" symptomatology, its arbitrary dividing lines between normalcy and pathology, and its cultural bias. African Americans, for example, are much more likely to earn the label of *psychotic* for the same behavior that elicits a milder *neurotic* label in whites,[42] but this had been the case long before the *DSM-5* hit the shelves.[43] The manual has also been accused of medicalizing human experiences that are not necessarily pathological. For example, under the *Diagnostic and Statistical Manual of Mental Disorders IV*, clinicians were advised not to diagnose major depression in people who had suffered the death of a loved one within the previous two months. But the *DSM-5* (the roman numerals were dropped after the fourth edition) has abandoned this bereavement exclusion, and many people take issue with treating the grief of the bereaved as a pathological condition. Some also criticize the book for reflecting the opinions of a closed circle of influential psychiatrists, and many are uncomfortable with the fact that it is used much more often in the United States than abroad.

There is little attention paid to addressing how profoundly culture affects the way mental disease appears within the *DSM*'s pages, and, as if all this weren't enough to hobble it as a tool, the text is also beholden to corporate and other financial interests, including pharmaceutical companies and the APA, which has raked in $100 million from its sales and licensing.[44]

However, the chief flaw of the *DSM*, from the perspective of this discussion of mental diseases caused by infection, is a key error of omission: despite the typically sluggish fourteen years of deliberation and voluminous documentation in which the authors of the newest revision indulged, the manual has maintained a perfect silence on what Ferris Jabr's 2013 *Scientific American* essay called "the biological underpinnings of mental disorders."[45]

Thus, although PANDAS is not a valid *DSM-5* disease category,[46] this signifies little. So the question remains: How do we determine whether the evidence that correlates infection with PANDAS rises to proof of causation? This issue applies not only to PANDAS but to all the possible links between infection and mental states that this book discusses.

Interrogating proof

The discovery of syphilis spirochetes in the brains of paretics struck the blinders from the eyes of the nineteenth-century doctors who treated those patients. The physicians produced detailed charts to document how often the disease and the paresis were associated and whether the syphilis seemed to precede the madness. What they emerged with was a correlation between the two disorders.

Yet approximately a century intervened between this correlation and the routine curing of paresis with antibiotics, which proved it was infectious. The change in treatment was the definitive indication that medicine had finally accepted the association between spirochetes and madness as a proven fact, but the slowness to translate that realization into practice is a drearily familiar scenario. Typically a very long lag time elapses between *Eureka!* and the acceptance of a new cause and treatment.

But how do we know when we have reached the eureka stage?

Despite the public's discomfort with infection as a cause of mental illness, it is a simple extension of the accepted nineteenth-century germ theory that posits infectious causes for a wide array of physical diseases. Should we not have to apply the standards set up by the architects of germ theory to establish proof? Can we?

In a word, no.

Basic standards for the proof of infectious-disease causation were laid down in 1883 by the German bacteriologists Robert Koch and Friedrich Loeffler, whose criteria came to be known as Koch's postulates. According to these, a suspected pathogen can be said to cause a disease only when (1) the germ is consistently associated with the disease; (2) it can be isolated from the sick organism and cultured; and (3) inoculating an organism with the pathogen should cause symptoms of the disease to appear. In 1905, another requirement was appended: The pathogen must be isolated again from the experimentally infected host.[47] However, at least one prominent researcher claims that only the first two postulates are Koch's and only they matter.[48]

Critics have invoked Koch's postulates to question the etiology of PANDAS and other madness caused by infection. But even in the nineteenth century, scientists realized the criteria's limitations; some microbes that caused disease failed to fulfill the postulates. Mary Mallon, dubbed Typhoid Mary, comes to mind; she was an asymptomatic carrier—that is, she carried the typhoid pathogen without suffering signs or symptoms of the disease herself—and similar carriers are found in cholera. This carrier scenario is so common in infectious disease, especially viral diseases such as polio, herpes simplex, and hepatitis C, as to invalidate Koch's first postulate. Polio causes paralysis in only a small number of infected people, yet we know polio is caused by the virus because the vaccine against poliomyelitis successfully prevents it.

Koch's second postulate rests on equally sandy ground, because some disease-causing microorganisms, such as prions, infectious proteins that many think responsible for Creutzfeldt-Jakob disease, cannot be grown in culture.

Koch himself knew that the third postulate was flawed; ever since the establishment of germ theory, it's been known that not all organisms exposed to a pathogen will fall ill. Immunological resistance, genetics, and variations of general health happen to them all. Noninfection may be due to such factors as having acquired immunity from previous exposures or vaccination.

Then, too, genetic immunity protects some; having an allele for Tay-Sachs confers some degree of immunity to tuberculosis, for example, and having sickle-cell trait does the same for some strains of malaria.[49] Perhaps this is why the third postulate specifies that the pathogen *should* cause symptoms, rather than that it *must*.

In short, the evidence tells us that Koch's postulates are sufficient—but not necessary—to establish causation.

Today, quite a few infectious agents are accepted as the cause of disease even though they do not fulfill Koch's postulates.[50] "We have to be ready to think of all sorts of new, clever ways to identify pathogens," says evolutionary biologist Paul Ewald, author of *The Evolution of Infectious Disease* and *Plague Time*. "We will have to abandon Koch's postulates in some cases."[51]

Arrowsmith in the twenty-first century

What, I wonder, does epidemiologist Ian Lipkin think? Like Dr. Martin Arrowsmith, the intrepid protagonist of Sinclair Lewis's 1925 novel *Arrowsmith,* Dr. Ian Lipkin is a peerless microbe hunter. He has identified hundreds of viruses, tracked pathogens from the Bronx to Beijing to Burundi, fingered West Nile virus as the cause of a mysterious 1999 encephalitis epidemic in New York City,[52] and advised the makers of the film *Contagion*. He knows a thing or two about linking infection to disease.

He also directs Columbia University's Center for Infection and Immunity, whose mission statement reads,

> We are committed to assembling a "global immune system" that will enable scientists and clinicians to manage potential threats before they can affect the health of communities worldwide.
>
> The first step toward achieving this goal is being able to quickly identify the pathogens that cause disease.

I arrive at Columbia's Mailman School of Public Health, just blocks from my former Harlem home, to ask Lipkin how his institute definitively fingers pathogens.

"It's nice to be back in Harlem," I volunteer to the affable security guard at the glassed-in front desk as I proffer my Columbia ID. I am quickly corrected. Peering closely at my card, he says, smiling, "This is *not* Harlem; it's Hamilton Heights." I return his smile, but nomenclature doesn't change the fact that I could throw rocks from here and hit no one but Harlemites; the university's medical enclave is nestled within it.

When I reach Lipkin's institute, however, I better understand the guard's distinction. The heart of the globe's immune system generates an ambiance that is light-years from the colorful urbanity surrounding it.

Everything looks gray, beige, or black. When the elevator reaches the seventeenth floor, the doors slide back smoothly, in silence, to reveal a capacious modern beehive housing workers in banks of identical desks; this is the anteroom of the center. As I step forward, their heads swivel briefly in response to this stranger among them; immediately, a neatly dressed young man walks over and politely questions me in hushed tones before ushering me past the first flank of podlike gray workspaces. There are no cubicle walls, and each desk is graced with a black phone, a charcoal-gray monitor, and a seated employee. I'm invited into a black ergonomic chair, where I sit alone and unregarded within the glassed-in conference room. Before me, the workers busily attend to their tasks in eerie silence; the conference room must be soundproofed.

A fifty-inch black monitor and a bone-colored spherical microphone depend from the ceiling, and a grayish keyboard and a few pages from an autism-study protocol are the only items on the table, which easily seats ten. It is made from the delicately varnished cross-section of a mammoth tree—rings, knots, and all—and it's the only object in sight that is visibly organic and that looks as if it could have been designed in the previous century. After twelve minutes, a young woman clad in dark gray and white opens the door, admitting a subdued hum of background activity. She utters my name, then wordlessly guides me down a corridor toward Ian Lipkin's inner office. It's adjacent to its own conference room, into which she motions me. I take a seat, and as she glides out of sight, I hear her announce to Lipkin: "Your ten o'clock."

I've been allotted twenty minutes. After a few of them pass, Lipkin enters, a slim man of average height who's fiftyish but looks a decade younger. He is wearing a pointed-collar cotton shirt of vaguely institutional green, neat, belted brown pants, rectangular bronze-rimmed glasses, and a moue of impatience. As we make eye contact, this changes to a small but pleasant smile that vanishes when he sees my extended hand. He demurs. "I don't shake hands, especially in winter."

"I understand," I say, because it's only logical behavior for a microbe hunter. He pauses and adds, awkwardly, "It's nothing personal," then slumps into his seat and stares at me with a dour expression.

There's little time, so I get right to it. "How do you prove causality in cases where you cannot apply Koch's postulates?"

Lipkin minces no words. "Koch's postulates are obsolete."

I point out that journal articles often invoke them as criteria.

"Well, they *sound* good, don't they?" he counters, raising an eyebrow and grinning. "But that's not the way you prove causation. Proof falls into three categories—the possible, the probable, and the definitive."

Lipkin deals in the definitive. "We've discovered more than five hundred viruses since I arrived at Columbia in 2002," including West Nile virus, which he identified as the cause of a North American encephalitis outbreak in 1999. Lipkin was the first to use high-throughput sequencing for pathogen discovery and he uses MassTag PCR and GreeneChip technology, two multiplex assays[53] that have identified and characterized his hundreds of viruses.

Moreover, Lipkin's work isn't limited to viruses. His empire of pathogen hunters investigates protozoa and fungi as well.

He's indicted inflammatory neuropathy in some ailments and shown that it can be treated with plasmapheresis. He's also shown that an infant's exposure to viral infections early in life changes the way his or her neurotransmitters function, suggesting a role for infections in schizophrenia and possibly autism.[54]

As he summarizes his team's protean achievements, I am pleasantly surprised by the witty and genial conversationalist who emerges. He even takes care to speak in accessible language; for example, he veers midphrase from "in vitro results" to "laboratory results" for clarity's sake. This isn't necessary, but it's thoughtful. I tell myself that his initial abruptness probably came of his being badly pressed for time; it must be hard to tear himself away from his well-oiled machinery of epidemiology, even for twenty minutes.

"I think that there are many examples where you cannot fulfill Koch's postulates," Lipkin continues. In those cases, what determines when something qualifies as proof? "There are the original Bradford Hill criteria, and other criteria people have talked about for years," Lipkin says, referring to Austin Bradford Hill, the English epidemiologist who suggested nine criteria for proof. They include *strength of association* (the larger the association, the greater the chance it is causal), *consistency of association*, and *biological gradient*, the idea that a greater number of exposures leads to a higher incidence of the effect. He also introduced the criterion of *plausibility*, stipulating that a believable mechanism must be proposed to tie cause to effect.

Plausibility. Believable. These words give me pause. Couldn't such a criterion exclude a true cause just because it isn't within one's habits of thought—that is, within the current paradigm that explains such illnesses? Dismissing a theory as unbelievable— scientists who were loath to admit that paresis was caused by the bacteria of syphilis did just this, as did physicians who refused to accept that pellagra was caused by a nutritional deficiency, not by an infectious disorder that was limited to blacks. Everyone "knew" that paresis was madness born of psychological causes and that pellagra was a racially bound disease of filth, so even in the face of definitive evidence to the contrary, some clung to these theories decades after they had been disproven. In other words, isn't the criterion of plausibility, in some cases, an invitation to cling to dogma?

Another Bradford Hill criterion seems even more problematic: *temporality*, which suggests that the effect must follow the putative cause closely in time. The infectious transmission of mental illness often transpires over a long interval that can obscure the cause-and-effect relationship. Paresis appears as long as three decades after an infection by *T. pallidum*, and influenza can trigger schizophrenia after twenty years. Rabies, however, can trigger madness within weeks or even days of infection, clarifying its connection to a precipitating animal bite. This makes the madness of rabies much easier to associate with infection, yet rabies, too, goes undiagnosed when months have intervened between an exposure and the onset of symptoms.

Koch's theory is also riddled with limitations. "Koch's postulates require that you grow something, put it in an animal model, and replicate disease," says Lipkin. "But there are agents that you can't cultivate in laboratories. You have infectious agents for which there is no animal model because you have to have a receptor for the virus," he explains. "Or you have to be able to grow the bacterium; all these things are difficult.[55] That's why we use what we describe as *possible, probable*, and *definitive* evidence of disease."

Possible means you have found an association. *Probable* incorporates such factors as location of the agent in the target tissues, levels of the pathogen or of antibodies to it, and biological plausibility. The ability to create animal models of diseases you are studying is key in establishing causality, Lipkin adds. "Do you have an analogous situation, and can you come up with a way of explaining it using an animal model that holds true?" he asks rhetorically.

"*Definitive* proof, which you may not get to for a while, means you have, one, satisfied Koch's postulates, or, two, demonstrated that introducing the vaccine reduces the incidence of disease or eliminates it completely, or that you have a specific drug that can improve the situation and that reduces the presence of the pathogen or antibodies," Lipkin summarizes. Just as the polio vaccine sharply reduced polio, researchers demonstrate the viral cause of an illness when they show that the vaccine against it lowers the frequency of disease.

"So there are three ways that you definitively prove something," continues Lipkin. "You prevent it with a vaccine; you treat it with a drug; or you go through Koch's postulates to identify the virus, grow it, then re-introduce it to replicate disease. But Koch's is an obsolete proof in an era of molecular markers."

Creatures of scientific habit

Two decades ago I was a visiting fellow at the Harvard School of Public Health. As a writer in residence at the Longwood medical complex in Boston, I learned a great deal about immunology, toxicology, psychiatric epidemiology, and medical writing. But intriguing, tacit elements of my education transpired outside of the classrooms and amphitheaters as I observed details ruling the social dynamics among researchers and physicians. I learned that the brilliant scientists and dedicated healers I observed were not always immune to illogic and could sometimes succumb to the same sort of biases as the rest of us.

I also learned that when all you have is a hammer, everything looks like a nail. Whether your tool of choice is an exhaustive command of genetics or an encyclopedic intimacy with

Freudian theory, it can became your preferred or even your default approach to medical problems, even after its limitations emerge.

Schizophrenia, for example, remains characterized as primarily genetic even though it has never been adequately explained by genetics. The mere 30 to 40 percent concordance of the disease in identical twins is testimony to this, as discussed in the previous chapter. Yet many cling to a purely genetic theory, which has become a dominant physiological paradigm for explaining disease rates and disparities, only recently tempered by epigenetics of the sort described in chapter 2. I recall that ascribing the disease to toxic family dynamics persisted long after theories of schizophrenogenic mothers and absent fathers had lost their credibility.

Scientists had fallen into a habit of paradigmatic thought, focusing on genetics, psychological trauma, and brain injury, all of which are implicated in schizophrenia but none of which completely explain the disease's prevalence. This habit made physical causes, like brain chemistry or even infection, less believable candidates.

In *The Structure of Scientific Revolutions*, Thomas Kuhn illuminates how introducing new knowledge that entails a shift in the prevailing paradigm evokes resistance and hostility to the new ideas. The hurdles are not always scientific, because all too often the mantle of science shrouds politics, social biases, and even petty jealousies that hamper the understanding of physical as well as mental diseases.

The concern, of course, is that science has sometimes been suppressed for nonscientific reasons—usually because it is politically inexpedient or it violates dogma or the tenets of the dominant belief systems.

I recall Kuhn's admonition as I notice that the word *controversial* in a journal article about PANDAS on Swedo's desk has been heavily circled in black. When I ask her about this, she shows she is quite alive to its semantic implications. Raising her eyebrows, she questions the rhetorical strategies of some critics: "They call PANDAS 'controversial,' but it is so only because certain people question its elements without understanding them, sometimes in contravention to the evidence. It's not aboveboard, but the very word conjures up a suggestion of...marginality, or of questionable science, without offering any specific criticism. It's just not logical."

I've heard the term *controversial* used in informal discussions and debates about the nature of PANDAS infections more often than in peer-reviewed journals. But it is also used in more accessible publications or sites such as Wikipedia, where laypeople and patients are likely to get their first exposure to PANDAS, an introduction that may be colored by such a loaded term. It implies skepticism in the same manner that the verb *claim* signals that a statement may be untrustworthy.

In 2005, Joanna Kempner of Rutgers University and her colleagues interviewed forty-one researchers about science that had been suppressed, and her team found that the manner in which such knowledge became marginalized and dismissed was "self-imposed, reflecting social, political, and cultural pressures on what is studied, how studies are performed, how data are interpreted, and how results are disseminated....We were surprised that respondents felt most affected by what we characterize as 'informal constraints.'" In other words, scientists who ventured into forbidden knowledge were often warned away from the topics by oblique disapproval from their colleagues that did not invoke scientific criteria and sometimes even descended to ad hominem attacks: "He's crazy," "He's not well thought of around here," and "That's controversial" are comments I heard when I asked academics about novel contested theories, from the role of the enteric nervous system in psychological disease to the flawed history of genetic theories of intelligence dissected by Stephen Jay Gould in *The Mismeasure of Man*. Such dismissals say nothing about the theory itself and everything about the theory's status as an acceptable area of study.

Spreading informally, forbidden knowledge demarcates some scientific territory as off-limits, Kempner wrote. "Researchers sometimes only know that they have encountered forbidden knowledge when their research breaches an unspoken rule and is identified as problematic by legislators, news agencies, activists, editors, or peers."[56] Scientists often choose to abandon the verboten topic or theory.

As researchers entertain the idea of infection as another root of mental disorders, we realize how often diseases, physical and mental, that have long been ascribed to genetics, diet, and behavior are actually infectious in nature. Acceptance has been hard and slow, and it's sometimes hampered not by scientific hurdles, but by social ones.

Hard-to-swallow proofs

Consider that until 1994, doctors told patients that their stress levels and diets—particularly their fondness for coffee and spicy foods—were causing their ulcers. Most physicians treated patients with acid control, prescribing not only Tagamet, which reduces stomach acid, but also bland diets and milk. (Except for a few mavericks, like John Lykoudis, a Greek practitioner who prescribed antibiotics in the 1950s and 1960s.) The milk and bland diets were only partially helpful, however, and so were supplemented by biofeedback and even psychological counseling, which did little to reduce the rates of peptic ulcer disease, or PUD.

However, in 1982 Australian physicians Robin Warren and Barry Marshall proved that *Helicobacter pylori,* a familiar bacteria living in our intestinal tracts, accounts for 90 percent of stomach and duodenal ulcers as well as for some other gastric diseases, including stomach cancer.

But wait: In 1982, *H. pylori* was discovered to cause most ulcers, so why did doctors continue to prescribe Tagamet and milk until 1994? And why does the medical literature show that Dr. John Lykoudis of Missolonghi, Greece, was curing ulcer patients with antibiotics as far back as 1958?

To find out, I perused the PubMed site for gastroenterology journals tracing ulcer treatment. I learned that during the century before Marshall and Warren's breakthrough, an infectious cause of ulcers had been "discovered" on least fifteen separate occasions by different clinicians.

More than a hundred and ten years ago, Professor Walery Jaworski of Krakow's Jagiellonian University described "spiral-shaped microbes in the human stomach" of his ulcer-plagued patients;[57] Giulio Bizzozero, a nineteenth-century Italian anatomist, had been the first to describe these troublemaking "corkscrew" bacteria in the stomach; and in the 1960s, Iranian surgeon Emami-Ahari saw evidence of bacterial infection in ulcers suffered by patients in his Tehran private clinic. He also used antibiotic therapy to cure them. These were just a few of the physicians who glimpsed the connection between gut pathogens and ulcers, although they didn't have the tools or intimacy with microbiology to specify *H. pylori* as the culprit. Nonplussed, I thought of Goethe, who wrote, "Everything has been thought of before, but the problem is to think of it again."

Lykoudis, however, took therapeutics a step further when he formulated a safe, effective antibiotic cocktail consisting of two quinolines, which are aromatic compounds with antibiotic qualities—the quinine used against malaria is one—and streptomycin, taken with oral vitamin A. In the heroic if not altogether wise tradition of physicians, he tested it on himself in 1958 and cured his own ulcers.[58] Calling his patented remedy

Elgaco,[59] formed from the words *elkos* (Greek for "ulcer"), *gastritis,* and *colitis,* he reported curing thirty thousand patients. Word spread quickly and new patients thronged his office, but the Athens Medical Association responded by denouncing Lykoudis as a huckster and fining him four thousand drachmas. The Greek government quickly followed suit, censuring and fining him for using Elgaco without the proper testing.[60]

The government's accusation was true, Lykoudis retorted, but he hadn't tested it because pharmaceutical companies had flatly refused to run studies of his controversial treatment. Lykoudis did not have the advanced training and expertise that would allow him to identify the organism that caused ulcers, but testing by others who did might have helped him amass an airtight case for infection. No university or company he approached was willing to do so, however.[61] He felt unfairly marginalized and persecuted by the medical establishment and the government alike. Was he? In retrospect, it seems likely. "No science is immune to the infection of politics and the corruption of power," wrote Jacob Bronowski, a Polish biologist, historian of science, and poet. Lykoudis and his shunned cure could have been Bronowski's poster child. In 1966, *JAMA* refused to publish the Greek physician's paper entitled "Ulcer of the Stomach and Duodenum," which outlined the link between infection and ulcers. With the exception of a self-published pamphlet, none of his writings on the subject ever found a publisher, ensuring that physicians the world over would cling to their prescriptions of Tagamet and milk.[62]

A century of resistance to accepting or even discussing and testing the role of bacteria in ulcers[63] made that relationship forbidden knowledge. The point is not that the dissenters were correct and the conventional practitioners were wrong; many would-be scientific innovators blame medical intolerance for their obscurity when that is not the case. Some are simply misguided, and still others are outright quacks and charlatans who decry the hostility of the medical establishment and compare themselves to Galileo and Semmelweis as they line their pockets with the fees of the gullible.

The real point is the *nature* of the refutation offered by the medical establishment. Rejection of Lykoudis's theory should have been based on science, data, evidence, and logic. When resistance to change is instead based on factors such as personality, bias, academic snobbery, political considerations, and a conspiracy of silence that ignores uncomfortable theories, the question becomes, as Lykoudis plaintively wrote, "Why the refusal even to test it?"

Without scientific publication or rigorous testing, the infection theory of ulcers was consigned to the forgotten annals of forbidden knowledge. Lykoudis's notebooks detail a life blighted by professional frustration; he died in 1980, just two years before Warren and Marshall validated his life's work.

The duo could prove the connection because they had access to tools unknown to Lykoudis, including the flexible fiber-optic endoscope developed in the late 1970s, which provided a safe technique to view the stomach and collect specimens from the gastric mucosa of live patients for more accurate diagnosis. Modern nutrient media and incubation techniques also allowed Warren and Marshall to grow the organisms in culture, as Koch and his scientific progeny dictate.

In 1985, having satisfied Koch's postulates, Warren and Marshall triumphantly published their findings that *H. pylori*, not stress and spices, causes ulcers. But once again, the *H. pylori* hypothesis failed to change physicians' behavior. According to the CDC, at that time, most physicians knew of the *H. pylori* association, but half of primary care doctors did not test their ulcer patients for *H. pylori*.[64] They ignored it while doling out treatments like acid suppressants, which were ineffective against the root cause of the disease. Despite their superior tools and access to publication, Warren and Marshall were about to share Lykoudis's professional fate: studied indifference and obscurity.

"Everyone knew that bacteria couldn't survive in the stomach's acid environment," Marshall told the *Sydney Morning Herald* to explain the widespread resistance to the discovery. "They'd been taught so at medical school."[65] In the end, it took more than scientific evidence to get the medical world's attention; it took showmanship. The same self-experimentation that Lykoudis had conducted privately, Marshall shrugged off his lab coat and his gravitas and performed publicly.

To illustrate his claim, Marshall drank a beaker of *H. pylori* in culture[66] in 1984, and within days, he was rewarded by nausea and vomiting. An endoscopy revealed the appearance of both *H. pylori* and gastritis, which Marshall was then able to banish with antibiotics. The fading of his symptoms in two weeks demonstrated, for at least the fifteenth time, that a microbe can cause gastric woes and that antibiotics can cure them.

In 1985 the victorious pair published their results in a wildly popular *Australian Medical Journal* paper, and in 1994, *JAMA* followed up with a National Institutes of Health consensus opinion that most duodenal and gastric ulcers were caused by *H. pylori* and that antibiotics were now the recommended treatment.[67] It turned out that milk and Tagamet had enjoyed their limited success only because lowering the stomach's acidity changed the stomach milieu sufficiently to discourage *H. pylori* infection.

The infectious cause of ulcers finally entered the medical canon when, in 1997, the Centers for Disease Control and Prevention spearheaded a public-health campaign to spread the word that ulcers were a curable infection, and in 2005 Marshall and Warren scored the ultimate validation: they were awarded the Nobel Prize in Physiology or Medicine for their "discovery of the bacterium *Helicobacter pylori* and its role in gastritis and peptic ulcer disease." Today we understand that ulcers are caused by *H. pylori,* spread by contaminated food and groundwater and through human saliva via kissing.[68]

Such mischaracterizations of microbial disease abound in history.[69] In nineteenth-century Florence, for example, Italian physician Domenico Antonio Rigoni-Stern noticed that cervical cancer affected married women and prostitutes[70] but spared nuns. His conclusion: Cervical cancer was caused by tight corsets.[71]

By the end of the Victorian era, women's doctors tied cervical cancer to early and frequent sexual contact with multiple partners—and to poor male hygiene. In the mid-nineteenth century, Alabama women's doctor James Marion Sims infamously declared that due to black women's lasciviousness, 60 percent of the black female patients seen in hospitals had cervical cancer. Cardiologist Daniel Hale Williams challenged his evidence, or rather the lack thereof, wondering in print how Sims could have determined this when he could produce no records, and black women were rarely permitted into the white hospitals of the time.[72] Still, Sims's views were widely adopted. By the 1970s, cervical cancer was laid at the doorstep of the sexual villain of the day: herpes infection. It was not until the 1980s that Harald zur Hausen finally discerned that strains 16 and 18 of the human papillomavirus, HPV, accompanied most cervical cancers and theorized that HPV was the cause in 70 percent of cases.

Only then could a vaccine against a major source of cervical cancer be crafted. It worked, demonstrating that HPV causes cervical cancer, for which zur Hausen won the 2008 Nobel Prize in Physiology or Medicine. For HPV, cancer is a strategy. Because sexual transmission of HPV is inefficient except in the most active and promiscuous individuals, the virus would have few chances to spread to another host if HPV strains did not trigger the cells they infect to continuously and recklessly divide—the definition of cancer—allowing HPV to divide and proliferate right along with them. The virus remains shrouded from surveillance by the immune system. Cancer is thus a means to an end, and once again the health of the human host becomes collateral damage.

In yet another example, heart disease has been especially riddled with stubborn mythology, including psychological determinism, a subtle form of blaming the victim, as the hostility and aggressive behavior of people with type A personalities was broadly indicted in heart attacks. We now know that infectious agents such as *C. pneumoniae* are key players that triple the risk of coronary artery disease. Stanley Prusiner's theory that infectious proteins caused both mad cow disease and its human variant, CJD, was met with hostility and ad hominem attacks. He was reviled as a self-promoting huckster for decades before winning the Nobel Prize for discovering the prion.

Resistance to discussing and testing the role of microbes in ulcers, heart disease, and cervical cancer transformed those relationships into forbidden knowledge. The pertinent question is not whether the theory is correct, but why the nature of the criticism leveled at it is informal and nonscientific or, in other cases, why the theory is ignored, guaranteeing it will be forgotten. Why does science treat some theories as taboo and forbid objective discussion and testing?

Certainly, compelling evidence is necessary before we change our thinking about the infectious transmission of diseases that were once "known" to have noninfectious causes. But definitive data is not always enough, because often, once it is presented, the evidence is ignored.

Even proven theories and demonstrated facts sometimes become forbidden knowledge, for social and political reasons as well as scientific ones. Such knowledge can be unacceptable for many reasons—it may call the theories or work of other scientists into question, or it may sabotage established hierarchies or an entrenched scheme of thinking about disease.

Sometimes the new paradigm exposes treatments as illogical and ineffective, and always, it does little to bolster the egos of scientists whose careers depend on subscribing to established disease paradigms. Although science is shaped by formal regulations and policies, researchers who traced its genesis found that, according to respondents, most of its constraints are informal or self-imposed, reflecting social, political, and cultural pressures on what is studied, how studies are performed, how data are interpreted, and how results are disseminated.

Discovering the roots of Tourette's and anorexia in sore throats is far from the strangest paradigm shift along the infection-and-mental-disease spectrum. There is also the case of mental disorders such as depression and autism that are cued by the microbes of the "second brain"—the one that resides in your gut, as the next chapter explains.

CHAPTER 4

Gut Feelings: The Brain in Your Belly

We have met the enemy, and he is us.

—*POGO* COMIC STRIP, 1971

Jeroen Raes glides onto the stage, all Dutch height and unhurried manner. Clad in a simple dark sweater but wearing confidence like an Armani suit, he glances at the overhead projection of his first slide before his gaze flits briefly in the direction of his audience. It doesn't alight there; he's unconcerned with eye contact.

"So you think you are human," he begins.

Raes is giving a Brussels TED talk about his work as director of Flanders's Vlaams Instituut voor Biotechnologie, or VIB, *the* Belgian research institute, and he tosses a dizzying array of numbers at us: "There are seven billion people on this planet," he announces, and goes on to say that our bodies are home to ten times as many microbial cells as human cells. My attention begins to wander, because I've heard these numbers before. Except for one.

"You know how many microbes there are [on earth]? Five nonillion."

Five nonillion? That's a 5 followed by 30 zeros. There are, in other words, as many microbes living on this planet as there are stars in the universe—multiplied by five million.

It's a good thing that the scientists in Paul de Kruif's *Microbe*

Hunters didn't know this. Even those irrepressible twentieth-century stalwarts might have despaired of exterminating their targeted pathogens had they known the size of the army arrayed against them. Instead, to a man — and they were all men — they were confident, even arrogant in their dominance. De Kruif presents them as conquering heroes of the microbial world, and his book is studded with martial metaphors, as are others of the genre — his *Hunger Fighters* and Han Zinsser's *Rats, Lice and History*. The warlike tone is echoed in the work of evolutionary theorists like George C. Williams, who wrote, "Natural selection, albeit stupid, is a story of unending arms races, slaughter and suffering."[1]

Casting the evolutionary contest as a war to the death between humans and microbes has become a cliché, reflected in the ways we conceptualize and speak about illness. Man fights to annihilate pathogens and vanquish disease. Microbes, although versatile, often favor guerrilla warfare, invading by stealth, crippling or taking over their hosts' immunological armies, and sapping their strength, blood, fluids, and resources before wiping them out. Patients "battle" cancer and drugs "suppress" infection in a scorched-earth arms race in which pathogens seek to eradicate their enemies by ever-harsher measures. And in this age of antibiotic-resistant organisms, we do the same to them. A type of bacterium has become drug resistant? Turn to a harsher antibiotic with a broader spectrum that will kill even more types — and render itself useless when bacteria become resistant to it too. Douse the environment, and yourself, for good measure, with the antimicrobial hand sanitizers that sprout on office walls, in restrooms, and inside handbags, although studies show that soap and water is more effective at keeping germs at bay without fostering dreaded resistant strains.

When we habitually describe contests between rival organisms as brute death matches, it helps such blunt and shortsighted approaches sound more rational and necessary than they are.

Influenced by Williams's 1960 book *Adaptation and Natural Selection,* the 1976 bestseller *The Selfish Gene* by Richard Dawkins moved this conflict squarely into the genetic arena by proposing that it is our species' genes, not our individual selves, that direct and profit from the battle for survival with the sole goal of propelling human genes into the next generation. We, apparently, are just along for the ride.

Dawkins's gene-centered view of evolution recasts many instances of apparent altruism as ruthless strivings for absolute dominance. When the monkey shares his meager meal with his community, when a woman risks her life to free her trapped cousin from a burning building, when a gay man helps support and raise his niece, the altruism does not seem to improve the altruists' fates. But, Dawkins argues, it is the gene that seeks immortality, so the more closely two individuals are genetically related, the more logical it is to behave selflessly. The fitness of the gene—that is, the extent to which it survives into the next generation—is the true measure of its evolutionary success, so saving the life of your relation, feeding your extended family from which you or your children will choose a mate, and ensuring that children who are genetically related to you survive all boost your genes' evolutionary fitness and are therefore sound survival strategies for your genome.

But despite the sophistication of these arguments, Dawkins perpetuated the military *Weltanschauung* when he invested the gene with the same anthropomorphic selfishness.

The microbes within

What if this worldview is wrong, and human evolutionary survival depends on something other than killing the competition in order to usher our genes safely into the future? What if, despite the rampant sickness caused by pathogens, our myopic view of them causes us to see malevolent foreign invaders where there are none and encourages us to obliterate organisms when our future health demands a more nuanced approach?

And what if, as the *Pogo* epigraph above suggests, the enemy is not wholly external?

For we are mostly microbes, and this is what Raes meant by his intimation that you are not wholly human. The numbers he offered supply evidence.

One hundred *trillion* viruses, fungi, archaea, and protozoa—but mostly bacteria—call your intestines home, and your guests outnumber your human cells ten to one. A coat of many microbes covers your skin, eyes, genitals, and mouth, each bacterial genotype specializing in an area of the body. Microbial scientists call this the *commensal microbiome*, a bit of a misnomer because the adjective describes a relationship in which one organism benefits while the other is unaffected, and as we shall soon see, you and your fellow travelers affect each other in many ways, sometimes dramatically.

Staphylococci colonize the skin, *Escherichia coli* prefer the colon, and lactobacilli coat the vagina. And that's just on the surface; ten thousand different species of organisms thickly populate your gut, the folded, invaginated, nine-meter expanse from your mouth through your stomach and anus. Just as our genes constitute our genomes, these creatures make up our microbiomes. But unlike genes, with their numerical constancy, the human microbiome is constantly changing in type and numbers. Its makeup varies in different sites of the body and often in different sites on the globe. It changes over a person's lifetime and in relation to the host's genes. And mental health changes with it.

"Half of your stool is not leftover food. It is microbial biomass," Lita Proctor, program director of the Human Microbiome Project, told the *New York Times*. We are so much larger than our microbial hangers-on that they contribute only an extra five or six pounds of body weight,[2] but like unemployed houseguests, you can never get rid of them.

Our wealth of internal life should not surprise us. In sheer numbers, microbes rule the world: every teaspoon of seawater contains five million bacteria and fifty million viruses,[3] which are the most numerous "living" things in the sea, a summit they reached by infecting other organisms, including bacteria.

Yet size and census counts matter less to our mental health than the microbiome's astonishing power to keep a person healthy—or ill—and guide the immune system's development. Embedded within the walls of your gut's microbial rain forest is a web that has a thousand times more neurons than your brain. This neural web of cells, dubbed the enteric nervous system, or ENS, weighs twice what your brain does and deploys neurotransmitters that communicate with the brain.

The ENS influences your mind as well as your body. It first does so by globally shaping the development of the immune system, 80 percent of whose cells reside in your gut.[4] By so guiding the immune system, the ENS determines your reaction to microbes' behavior and how the interplay of the immune system and microbes affects your health, both physical and mental. But evidence from human studies suggests that the ENS is also directly connected to some specific mental disorders, including depression, autism, and possibly chronic fatigue syndrome. This explains why electrical stimulation of the vagus nerve, for example, is a treatment for depression.[5] "I'm always by profession a skeptic," Dr. Emeran Mayer, professor of medicine and psychiatry at the University of California, Los Angeles, told NPR, "But I do believe that our gut microbes affect what goes on in our brains."[6]

Semantics shape conception, so in order to understand how the enteric microbes and the ENS direct the formation of our immune systems, it helps if we take off the verbal blinders. The warlike metaphors of which science is so fond distort our view and limit our ability to express what is happening, as a type of "war cam" disregards mutualism, symbiosis, and the many benefits that microbes impart. Martial language fosters a myopia that shrouds the true nature of our intimate relations with some bacteria.

Rather than mounting direct attacks on the body's immune system and brain, as the traditional language of *battling* and *vanquishing* microbes assumes, the internal microbiome subtly shapes and directs immune responses and, therefore, health and behaviors. As I'll soon explain, despite our big, complex brains, our single-celled passengers have a disquieting ability to manipulate us. And although this can evoke discomfort, it can also be a good thing.

Passengers is not quite the correct term. Most of the human bacterial complement has lived and evolved with our species for more than eight hundred million years,[7] and some have melded so intimately with our bodies that they literally have become us.

For example, each human cell contains critically important organelles called mitochondria. They process food into energy-rich *adenosine triphosphate*, or ATP, molecules, whose high-energy bonds provide 90 percent of the fuel that we need to function. A mitochondrion is an endosymbiont (from the Greek words for "within," "together," and "living"), an organism that lives within the cell or body of another organism.

Widely accepted endosymbiotic theory holds that eons ago, these mitochondria were free-living bacteria that found it in their evolutionary interests to move into human cells permanently. As they became an essential part of us, we benefited as well, from those high-energy ATP bonds. There is plenty of evidence of mitochondria's bacterial origins: mitochondria reproduce by dividing, as bacteria do, and they have even retained their own thirty-seven genes contained in the circular single-stranded molecule of DNA that is typical of free-living bacteria but that we now count among our human genes. More than thirteen diseases are caused by mutations in these mitochondrial genes, including forms of diabetes and deafness that are inherited through our mothers,[8] but eliminating mitochondria is not an option, because we cannot survive without them.

There are many other types of relationships between us as hosts and our resident microbes that are often broadly characterized as *symbiosis* or *commensalism,* describing a relationship in which at least one of the organisms benefits. In *mutualism,* both organisms benefit.

We are home to other endosymbionts. We need the stomach bacteria that stimulate our immune-system development, digest our fibrous foods, and unlock nutrients like isothiocyanate, which protects against cancer and is extracted from the broccoli we eat. Microbes neutralize external pathogens, like the ingested bacteria that cause food poisoning. We need the resident microbes that make vitamins such as biotin, vitamin K,[9] and vitamin D,[10] and we may even need *Helicobacter pylori,* which causes ulcers and stomach cancers but seems to sometimes protect against obesity. Bacteria also are necessary for metabolizing drugs, and how much of some medications, like the heart drug digoxin, reaches a person's bloodstream depends on which bacteria are in his microbiome.[11]

No wonder microbial scientists are wont to refer to the organisms in the microbiome as our "friends." Jeroen Raes's work at VIB[12] includes experiments that show how anxiety behavior and exploratory behavior in mice are determined by what flora they have, and Dr. Ramnik Joseph Xavier, director of the Center for the Study of Inflammatory Bowel Disease at Harvard Medical School, agrees. Xavier points out that we rely on microbes for the folic acid that is essential to health and necessary to prevent birth defects. He warns against using probiotic supplements to do this job, because they introduce too few microbes and are not within the intestines' carefully curated right balance: "Bacteria survive and do better when they are with their friends."

Raes and his team divined the numbers he bandies about by using techniques unknown to the twentieth-century microbe hunters. They extracted DNA from the microbes in our internal rain forest using automated sequencing machines to determine how many and what kinds of microbes are resident in both healthy and diseased guts. They then assessed what these microbes' genes did, because microbes other than mitochondria have genes too, a lot of them. When a European Union consortium assessed the genomes of 124 people, it found that the microbes within each individual harbor 3.3 million different genes, dwarfing the mere 25,000 in the human genome.[13]

What, then, does it mean to speak of the human genome when we carry millions more bacterial genes than *Homo sapiens* genes? And if we speak of the medical fortunes of a selfish gene, can we separate our species' genes from those of the microbial multitudes that have evolved with us so closely and for so long that we now cannot live without them?

The wandering nerve

Human life is defined by this obligate friendship with trillions of bugs, but each of us begins life sterile and innocent of microbes within the selectively permeable space suit of the placenta. (Some question the placenta's sterility, but a 2014 *New York Times* article overstated the case when it claimed, "The finding [which suggests newborns may acquire much of their gut bacteria from the placenta] overturns the conventional wisdom that the placenta is sterile."[14] *Overturned* is premature; many microbiologists think that the placenta's small community of bacteria is not acquired until it traverses the vagina after delivery.[15])

But all agree that early in fetal development, the *neural crest,* a short-lived structure composed of pluripotent stem cells, differentiates into a rainbow of varied structures, including skin, muscle, heart, and fat tissue. The two poles of a person's neurological being also spring from the neural crest: the central nervous system, or CNS, which consists of the brain and spinal cord,[16] and the peripheral nervous system, including the ENS. Both contain neurons, neurotransmitters, and messenger proteins within a staggeringly complex circuitry, but they develop and function separately, with the ENS migrating to line the gut. As we will see, the CNS is the frequent target of neurotransmitters dispensed from microbes and implicated in mental disease.

As they develop, the two systems come to communicate through the vagus nerve, the tenth cranial nerve, whose long path meanders from the midbrain through the neck and chest before terminating in the peritoneal cavity. This path gives the nerve its name: *vagus* is Latin for "wandering."

After the fetus has developed for nine months, powerful uterine muscles propel the baby through his mother's birth canal, where he acquires her vaginal, fecal, and skin germs to emerge veiled in the microbial life that will determine his medical fate. Everything from the refinement of the skin and blood vessels to the development of the immune system is directed by such microbial anointings.[17]

As some microorganisms flourish and others die out, your gut becomes an evolutionary chessboard, courtesy of your developing immune system and your environmental exposures— including the diet that your mother chooses for you. Breast-fed babies acquire a distinctive microbial world that is far richer and populated with different species than the bottle-fed babies'. Breast-fed children benefit from exposure to the mother's immune defenses, while formula-swillers miss out on Mom's gastric lactobacilli and borrowed immunity.

During those first months and years of life, a person's exposure to antibiotics is fraught with lingering consequences. In mice, as in humans, antibiotics kill off some microbes while leaving others to thrive, and this changes the nature of the microbial community. If the antibiotics' collateral damage decimates the "wrong" bacteria, say *H. pylori*, which causes 90 percent of ulcers, the mouse will grow obese. If the antibiotics kill off a different set of bugs, the baby becomes more likely to develop allergies or asthma.[18]

Your enteric microbiome—the population of bacteria, viruses, and fungi in your gut and elsewhere—mutates constantly as a result of complex interactions that scientists are still unraveling. Meanwhile, the versatile vagus nerve, which connects the CNS and ENS, comes to manage many disparate functions such as heart rate, sweating, speaking, breathing, and coughing. It is even involved with the inner ear, which is why some people cough when the ear is tickled. The hardworking vagus also governs digestive functions such as peristalsis, the involuntary movements of the intestine that shepherd food along the gut.

It was through peristalsis that English physiologists William M. Bayliss and Ernest H. Starling first showed how the ENS functions independently of the brain. In 1899, the University College duo described how hormones were regulated in the gut. They discovered that applying pressure within the abdominal cavity of dogs triggered the "peristaltic reflex"—contractions followed by a propulsive wave that moves food through the stomach. In humans as well as dogs, these movements are necessary for digestion, but were they controlled by the ENS, or did the brain dictate them via the abdominal nerves? To find out, Bayliss and Starling boldly cut the Gordian knot, severing all the nerves connecting the brain and ENS. The peristalsis continued, demonstrating that the ENS governs it independently of the brain.

But rather than place the ENS on equal footing with the

brain, scientists simply subsumed the enteric nerves under the heading "parasympathetic nervous system" as brain studies focused on how neurotransmitters dictate mood and behavior. Not until 1967 did the ENS studies of Michael Gershon, now chairman of anatomy and cell biology at Columbia Presbyterian Medical Center, reveal the existence of the neurotransmitter serotonin in the ENS as well as in the brain.

In Aldous Huxley's *Brave New World,* the drug Soma provides contentment and euphoria. Such instant utopia seems chimerical and ethically questionable, but if there *were* a happiness drug, serotonin would be it. Neuroscientists think that it elevates mood and is crucial for emotional health and balance. Besides bolstering feelings of well-being, serotonin eases the function of the digestive system. And 90 percent of the body's serotonin emanates from the ENS, *not* the brain. Serotonin's usual target? The central nervous system. The neurotransmitters dopamine, glutamate, norepinephrine, and nitric oxide are also deployed by the gut, and 90 percent of vagal fibers carry information from the gut to the brain, not the other way around.[19] ENS pioneer Gershon, author of *The Second Brain,* followed his discovery with innovative research into how the ENS uses infectious agents to produce mood disorders and mental illness. Because the antidepressant medications called selective serotonin reuptake inhibitors (SSRIs) increase serotonin levels, it's little wonder that meds meant to cause chemical changes in the mind often provoke GI issues as a side effect. Irritable bowel syndrome—which afflicts more than two million Americans— also may arise in part from too much serotonin in our entrails and could perhaps be regarded as a casualty of the second brain.

Microbes affect the brain by activating the gut endocrine system, which produces neurotransmitters and related signaling molecules called neuropeptides. These chemicals are involved in social behaviors and in learning, memory, pain relief, reward, and food intake.

Gut feelings

Researchers must create animal models of disease that mirror human ailments or behaviors so the animals can stand in as test subjects when studies are too unwieldy or unethical to attempt in humans, and research laws and ethics generally require that animal studies precede similar testing in humans. Creating animal models of disease can be challenging, but mimicking human emotions and behaviors presents an even greater hurdle. How, for example, can you duplicate human anxiety, panic attacks, or hopelessness in mice?

Well, you could buy the emotions. Mice are bred and sold with inherited temperaments; for example, there are high-anxiety and low-anxiety stocks.

Or you could make your mice go swimming. Persistent anxiety and depression are often modeled and measured by a forced-swimming test called the *behavioral despair test* or *Porsolt forced-swimming test.*

Any neophyte swimmer who's sought to conquer a fear of the deep end can appreciate this classic model of murine anxiety and depression. A mouse is placed in a water-filled transparent acrylic swimming chamber from which it cannot escape and left there for fifteen minutes. It's then fished out, and after twenty-four hours, the mouse is subjected to another swimming test of five minutes. The time that it spends in this chamber without moving, called immobility time, is considered a measure of hopelessness.

This model seems far from perfect. Some consider applying the concept of despair to a mouse a troubling bit of anthropomorphism, and others question whether the period of immobility may represent not hopelessness but an attempt to conserve resources after the mouse learns that escape is impossible. However, mice that are given antidepressants swim for longer periods and more vigorously than controls, and scientists (and the makers of antidepressants) have chosen to accept this as a measure of alleviated depression and despair. So have immunologists who wish to learn how commensal microbes regulate complex behaviors like anxiety, learning, memory, and appetite.

Some microbes directly produce neuroactive molecules that affect brain function and have been used to treat autism symptoms in mice. Researchers raised mice that had no microbiomes, then seeded these germ-free mice with colonies of whatever organism they wished to study. When scientists gave such sterile mice the bacteria *Lactobacillus rhamnosus*, the mice showed fewer depressive behaviors in the swimming test. However, when they gave the *L. rhamnosus* and then severed the vagus nerve (and thus the ENS's connection to the brain), the mice were not soothed by the lactobacilli in the gut, so scientists concluded that *L. rhamnosus* helped govern depression and depressive behavior by activating the vagus nerve. Other bacteria produce natural antianxiety agents, such as an endogenous form of Valium, a benzodiazepine. In his book *Missing Microbes*, Martin J. Blaser points out that people who are dying of liver cancer often become comatose, but if they are given a drug that stops the action of this natural Valium, they awaken. This is because healthy livers can break down the natural benzodiazepines and prevent them from affecting mood and consciousness, but nonfunctioning livers cannot, and the endogenous benzodiazepines go directly to the brain, where they rob the patient of consciousness.[20]

Yet another type of bacterium was shown to protect against a murine version of multiple sclerosis. Mice that were infused with *Bacteroides fragilis* by Caltech neuroscientists became more resistant to multiple sclerosis, but only if a certain regulatory T cell, CD25, was active. If the action of CD25 was blocked, *Bacteroides fragilis* could not protect the mouse against MS.

But the most curious results, for our purposes, came when the bacterium *B. fragilis* was injected into so-called autistic mice.

A burgeoning of disease and distrust

In 1994, Joseph, my nephew, was five years old, a beautiful little boy with a warm, gentle demeanor and a distracted air.[21] But he didn't yet speak, and my brother and his wife had sought answers for this since he'd turned two. At that time, his hearing had been extensively tested and his intelligence called into question, but the source of his silence remained unclear. Now, three years later, they were left hanging with such airy platitudes as "Oh, he'll probably grow out of it."

This wasn't nearly good enough, and my brother began taking his son to see specialists, paying a small fortune for out-of-network consultations that quickly deteriorated. He and his wife were questioned extensively about their home environment in a manner that annoyed me, if not my brother. He was vigorously pursuing an answer in the face of medical indifference; the fact that he also had to suffer implications that he was somehow to blame seemed profoundly unjust.

In 1996, we learned that autism was what was wrong, and our family struggled to deal with the shock. The disease is characterized by atypical communication and language development, avoidance of eye contact, and sensory experiences that differ from the norm, which explained Joe's acute dislike of certain foods and textures. Aside from this, the disease was highly variable. We learned just enough to worry about Joe's future, but my brother, as is his wont, saw the bright side. "Now that he has the diagnosis, he'll qualify for medical treatment, special education, and services. Now I know I'll be able to care for my son."

Today my brother, who has divorced and remarried, is the

primary caregiver for Joe, a friendly, happy, and industrious high-school graduate in his twenties.

Around 1911, Swiss psychiatrist Eugen Bleuler coined the word *autistic* to describe what he called the "morbid self-admiration" shown by children with what was then regarded as a type of schizophrenia.[22] From the Latin *autismus*, meaning "self," the word reflects the inward focus of autistics. The term made its first appearance in the *Diagnostic and Statistical Manual of Mental Disorders* in 1980 as a type of schizophrenia, but by 2013 it occupied its own disease category, as autism spectrum disorder, or ASD, with conditions such as Asperger's subsumed. Autistic children were once hidden away, but today medicine recognizes that the right combination of support can give affected people a good quality of life. However, autism's frequency has exploded in a disturbing manner and the disorder has assumed center stage as people debate whether we are in an autism epidemic, and if so, why? According to the CDC, one of every sixty-eight U.S. children is diagnosed with ASD, a mushrooming of 30 percent since 2012,[23] and it is twenty times more common now than it was in the 1940s. The surge is not confined to the United States; Norway diagnoses six cases for every thousand children, a tenfold increase since the 1980s.[24] This increase in diagnosis is easily explained by a wider awareness of the disorder and better diagnostic tools, coupled with incentives such as the medical, educational, and financial support a child's diagnosis offers parents like my brother. Still, the dramatic increase in autism provides a case study in twenty-first-century medical anxiety. When it comes to the state of autism research, perhaps Professor Jeremy Nicholson of Imperial College London said it best: "We know a lot about autism, but we don't understand much." But an escalating number of cases abroad as well as in the United States feeds a sense of urgency.

The disease has spawned seemingly endless controversy,

beginning with the question of whether, despite its medical approbation, it is even a disease at all. In his revelatory book *Dread: How Fear and Fantasy Have Fueled Epidemics from the Black Death to Avian Flu,* epidemiologist Philip Alcabes dissects autism in the light of fears of modernity and observes that the furor over whether it is caused by immunizations obscures the possibility that we may not be dealing with a disease at all but rather a disquieting but normative human type.

There are precedents for creating a disease from a human outlier. Philosopher Ian Hacking notes early in his essay "Making Up People"[25] that "statistical analysis of classes of people is a fundamental engine. We constantly try to medicalise." And in "The Looping Effects of Human Kinds,"[26] he writes, "We engage in ways of classifying [people] that became possible only in industrial bureaucracies."

Some categories of people did not exist until society created them. Adolescents, perverts, people suffering from multiple personality disorder—these are kinds of people that did not inhabit preindustrial societies, at least not as any recognizable group. Since the nineteenth century, the human penchant for compartmentalization to deal with the stresses of modernity has impelled us to categorize people, partly to help them fit in.

We cannot be sure that autism has truly earned its disease label. But Alcabes, professor of public health at Adelphi University, makes a direct and practical observation in *Dread* that can hardly be refuted: debate over autism's cause deflects attention from the question of whether people who exhibit autism's symptoms are truly diseased. "The controversy over causes," he writes, "makes autism seem less like a broad spectrum of normative mental-emotional states and more like an illness.... The dialogue about the nature and origin of the epidemic helps create the epidemic."[27]

However, in a 2015 e-mail, Alcabes added that when writing *Dread* he was "uncertain whether there had really been a biological shift leading to more children who were quirky and unable to multitask, or if the epidemic was really just perceptual. I wrote the chapter in hopes of arguing for a more benign, de-pathologizing, way of looking at autism.... I'm more sure now that something really *has* changed biologically."

If some autism is caused by infection, this helps validate its disease status. Are there any microbial causes? Perhaps.

I earlier mentioned that *B. fragilis* protects against a type of multiple sclerosis in mice under certain conditions. The bacteria also address the communication deficits that are central to autism in mice. As revealed in chapter 2, the children of mothers who contract severe viral infections while pregnant have a higher risk of autism. Paul Patterson of Caltech created mice with autism using a viral mimic that evoked an immune response in the mouse mothers similar to the one you would see in real viral infections. The offspring of these mice displayed the basic behaviors associated with autism.

However, when *B. fragilis* was added to the gut of an autistic mouse, the microbes produced neuroactive molecules that are known to enhance social behavior, and the mouse's social interactions were enriched.[28] How did these beneficial bacteria get from the gut to the central nervous system in order to change behavior? In their 2013 *Cell* paper,[29] the investigators explain that the guts of the autistic mice were more permeable—"leaky"—which allowed neuroactive molecules to pass through the intestines into the bloodstream. Once there, they circulated to the brain and caused behavior changes.

Autism's clinical picture is quite variable and the disorder probably has many causes, but this leaky gut is more than a feature of autism; it can sometimes be the cause. Michael Gershon has discovered that the same genes involved in the formation of synapses (infinitesimal spaces between neurons where communication by neurotransmitters takes place) in the brain are also involved in the formation of ENS synapses. "If these genes are affected in autism," he says, "it could explain why so many kids with autism have GI motor abnormalities" as well as elevated levels of serotonin.[30]

It's not completely surprising that interactions between the gut and immune system affect our thinking, feelings, and behavior; our language suggests that we've long sensed this. At my college and many others, students jubilantly recommended easy, intuitive courses to each other as "gut" courses, implying that little toil was needed because visceral wisdom would get you through without much studying. John Wilce, Ohio State coach, physician, and university professor, coined the phrase *intestinal fortitude* around 1915. It means "courage, willpower, guts, stamina, and determination."[31] Who has not endured loss of appetite, stomach cramps, or butterflies when facing a confrontation, an important test, or—*quelle horreur*—public speaking? Our instincts tell us that knowledge, fear, and courage emanate from the gut. But until recently, determining precisely how was difficult, because most gut microbes could not be cultured and studied in the laboratory.

We've long known that stress and fear produce gastrointestinal pyrotechnics, but in 1933 neuropathologist Armando Ferraro and clinical psychiatrist Joseph E. Kilman turned the equation on its head when they posited in *Psychiatric Quarterly* "the existence of cases of mental disorders which have as a basic etiological factor a toxic condition arising in the gastrointestinal tract."[32]

The duo, based at the New York Psychiatric Institute, theorized that some mental illnesses arose from differences or changes in the permeability of the gut that permitted potentially harmful chemicals to leak from it. Sometimes these chemicals combined in a fearful synergy. They then made their way to the CNS, where they were much more toxic at relatively low levels than they were in the gut. Once in the CNS, they caused serious destruction. Researchers called this effect *autointoxication genera.*[33]

The results, proposed Ferraro and Kilman, were legion: levels of inflammatory cytokines increased, and microbes produced more or fewer neurotransmitters, causing levels to rise or fall alarmingly, all of which could lead to depressed or anxious moods. This situation was worsened by the fact that intestinal microbiota would normally attempt to counteract the surges of neurotransmitters by releasing cytokines that added to the witches' brew from the leaky gut.

A person's behavior can be transformed by levels of cytokines that are too low to detect by conventional tools, which makes identifying the responsible microbes very difficult.[34]

Autism's leaky origins

Normally the tubes and pouches of the digestive system are surrounded by an impermeable wall of cells that protect the abdominal cavity from the stomach's sea of gastric acid, and the neurons of the central nervous system from the microbes of the gut and their psychoactive products. But when a medical condition or other event causes a break or weakening of this wall, dangerous substances, including pathogens, can leak through it and enter the bloodstream. The breach may be caused by something as ominous as HIV infection or alcohol abuse, or it can be the product of inflammatory bowel disease (IBD) or autoimmune disorders. It may occur after radiation therapy, stress, exhaustion, or severe allergic reactions to food. Regular use of seemingly innocuous medications like OTC painkillers and antibiotics can also compromise the intestinal walls and cause a leaky gut. What's more, reverse causation is a possibility, because a leaky gut can also *cause* some cases of IBD and autoimmune disorders. And some researchers think that the atypical, late-onset form of autism may be due to the leaky-gut syndrome, theorizing that mental diseases such as depression, like autism, are sometimes caused by microbes, psychoactive molecules, and toxic substances that slip from the viscera and migrate to the brain. In a study of depressed people that appeared in the May 2013 issue of *Acta Psychiatrica Scandinavica,* 35 percent of subjects showed serological evidence of leaky gut.[35] This condition is currently being successfully treated with a combination of glutamine, *N*-acetylcysteine, and zinc—all believed to have anti-inflammatory properties—in the relatively few cases that are diagnosed. The diagnosis is gaining traction in the wake of such research, but we cannot yet be sure of the causal connection.

The science and ethics of vaccination in the context of autism fears have been exhaustively debated elsewhere, most recently in Eula Biss's fine 2014 book *On Immunity: An Inoculation,* and I must forgo adding much to the discussion because it ranges almost completely outside the scope of this book, which focuses on infectious triggers of mental disorders.

Almost completely—there is an exception. In June 2010, Jeremy Nicholson of Imperial College London undertook human studies of the microbiome's role in autism. He investigated the intestinal "forests" of thirty-nine children with autism and found that, unlike their twenty-eight nonautistic siblings and a control group of thirty-four unrelated children without autism, those with autism showed changes in their gut bacteria,[36] suggesting that in some cases, autism may result from such changes.

The symptoms of autism usually appear during infancy or early childhood, although they are not always recognized as such until later, as in the case of my nephew. A 2010 study[37] found that a group of six-month-olds displayed similar behavior when it came to gazing at faces, sharing smiles, and vocalizations, but by the time the children were a year old, those who went on to develop autism had largely lost these behaviors.

Other parents report that their autistic children seemed to develop normally until later, about age three, at which point the features of autism suddenly appeared. Parents of children who have what's called "regressive-onset" autism often report that symptoms began after their child was given antibiotics that were followed by persistent diarrhea.

Proponents of the regressive-onset theory suggest that the antibiotics selectively kill some microbes, and as the community of microbes in the bowels of these children changes, it becomes colonized by bacteria that produce toxins that harm neurons, bringing on the symptoms of autism.

These troublemaking bacteria wear coats of lipopolysaccharides, or LPS, a tongue-twisting name for molecules that contain antigens and that elicit strong immune responses in animals. These LPS produce endotoxins, poisons that bacteria normally retain within their cell walls.[38]

The endotoxin-covered bacteria have evolved to be adept at *crypsis;* that is, the ability to escape detection by other organisms. In this case, the bacteria avoid destruction by the immune system by adopting a wily camouflage. On their surface, they present portions of their endotoxins that chemically resemble molecules on human cells, masking their true identity and fooling the immune system into thinking that LPS are a nonthreatening part of the host's self. This strategy is called *molecular mimicry.* In this theory of the origin of autism, the LPS-clad bacteria proceed to exude their poisons, the affected neurons become impaired or die, and the symptoms of autism emerge.

Finding an animal whose reaction to the LPS-veiled bacteria resembles that of humans would seem the logical next step for testing this theory, but rodents make dodgy models for studying the effects of endotoxins because humans are far more sensitive to them. Ingesting one microgram—that's one millionth of a gram—for every kilogram of body weight will send a person into shock, but mice tolerate a thousand times that dose without ill effects.

Happily, human studies have been conducted to test the theory. When the stools of children were analyzed, those of children with regressive-onset autism had much greater numbers of clostridium bacteria, which thrive when antibiotics kill other species in the bowel. In addition, compared to controls, a greater-than-usual diversity of clostridium proliferated.[39]

There are many infamously toxic strains of clostridium, from *C. difficile,* which causes diarrhea and sometimes colitis in the aftermath of antibiotics, to *C. botulinum,* which causes fatal food poisoning but has been tamed for cosmetic use as Botox, to *C. tetani,* which causes the equally fatal tetanus. Another member of the genus, *C. perfringens,* causes gas gangrene. What all these species of clostridium have in common is that they produce a dizzying assortment of toxins that attack neurons, and by doing so, they encourage madness as well as death.

In another study of children with regressive-onset autism following antibiotics and chronic diarrhea, ten children were given the antibiotic vancomycin by mouth.[40] If this routed the clostridium and cured the symptoms of autism, the recovery would serve as evidence that the clostridium levels were associated with the autism. Before and after the children were given the vancomycin, their skills and behaviors were evaluated in several ways, including by clinical psychologists who viewed videotapes of children but did not know who had been treated.

The scores revealed that eight of ten children demonstrated improvement after being on vancomycin. Although the response was not long-lasting, this points to a new treatment direction.

It's important to note that this study did not suggest that the initial use of antibiotics caused autistic symptoms, only that these symptoms were correlated with changes in the gut. It's possible that parents' belief in antibiotic-triggered symptoms is a result of recall bias. Or parents may unwittingly exaggerate the proximity of antibiotic administration and symptoms.

And not everyone agrees that regressive-onset autism even exists. Some insist that these children had not developed normally, but that their deficits and missed milestones had gone unnoticed until the other symptoms of autism emerged.

Even if larger future studies validate the finding that microbial changes are causally related to some types of autism, this is *not* an argument against using antibiotic therapy, which is often necessary and lifesaving, during childhood. Before such treatment was available, diseases killed and incapacitated children in numbers far greater than those who may risk late-onset autism. It may, however, be yet another argument for using more specific antibiotics to avoid changing the incredibly complex microbiome more than is necessary, as chapter 7 discusses.

Microbial frenemy

Helicobacter pylori, found in 90 percent of people with ulcers and stomach cancers, wreaks even greater havoc when it escapes from the gut. According to a report in *Psychosomatic Medicine*, errant *H. pylori* also contributes to the cognitive impairment of Alzheimer's disease. People who are infected with *H. pylori* perform significantly worse on cognitive tests than those who are uninfected, writes the study's coauthor May Baydoun. Her laboratory found that *H. pylori* cells travel from the gut to the brain, where the bacterial cells aggregate with the characteristic amyloid proteins of Alzheimer's and trigger the buildup of plaque. Baydoun, a scientist at the National Institute on Aging, estimates that about 20 percent of people younger than forty and half of adults older than sixty are infected with *H. pylori*.[41]

Worse, the bacteria's effects may not be limited to aging

brains; children infected with this ulcer-causing bacteria performed more poorly than controls on IQ tests in a study that suggests a broader link between *H. pylori* infection and cognitive impairment. *H. pylori* can be eliminated with antibiotics, which might conceivably lower the incidence or severity of Alzheimer's, but this is a move to ponder carefully, because the pathogen has beneficial effects as well. The bacteria's decline coincides with the epidemic of obesity and diabetes in developed countries. Josep Bassaganya-Riera conducted *H. pylori* studies that suggested this maligned catalyst of ulcers, stomach cancer, and cognitive erosion acted as bacterial armor against obesity. His laboratory at Virginia Tech's Center for Modeling Immunity to Enteric Pathogens is where, he says, "we demonstrated for the first time that gastric colonization with *H. pylori* exerts beneficial effects in mouse models of obesity and diabetes."

Other constituents of the microbiome have positive effects on mood and mental health. Lactobacillus, for example, seems to bestow serenity. Healthy human volunteers who consumed a mix of *Lactobacillus helveticus* and *Bifidobacterium longum* exhibited less anxiety and depression, while students' stools contained fewer lactobacilli during a high-stress exam period than during a less stressful period. These findings suggest an inverse link between stress and lactobacilli that will need to be more fully investigated.

Preparations containing lactobacilli and other probiotic microbes are often touted and sold as health supplements that can improve everything from mood to digestion, but scientists like Ramnik Xavier advise caution. Some of the commercial claims are unproven, warns Xavier, and the microbes may not be helpful when isolated from their companion organisms or when taken by people who do not suffer from leaky-gut syndrome.

One group of investigators scrutinized probiotics to see which, if any, might exploit the benefits of the ENS rather than the credulousness of consumers, and their 2007 report on preliminary human studies, published in the *European Journal of Clinical Nutrition,* demonstrated that consuming some probiotic strains can improve cognition and mental outlook via the psychotropic influence of lactobacillus and bifidobacterium. In an intriguing grace note, their work mentions why honey is so soothing: kynurenic acid,[42] which is produced by intestinal microbiota but also found in honey, is easily absorbed from the intestines and is an anxiolytic, defusing anxiety by damping the activity of excitatory amino acid receptors. Certain vegetables contain kynurenic acid too, but tubers and greens stirred into that comforting cup of tea sounds far less inviting.[43]

Know thyself: The Human Microbiome Project

Our bacterial genes outnumber our human genes by an order of magnitude,[44] and bacterial cells outnumber our human ones ten to one. After beginning life wholly human, we soon become 90 percent microbial. What picture of our health, including our mental health, can emerge without knowing something of the microbes within?

In 2007 the federal government sought to help microbiologists untangle the complexity of the microbial biome when it committed $115 million to the Human Microbiome Project, or HMP,[45] which is to culminate in 2015.[46] In a parallel to the Human Genome Project, two hundred scientists at eighty institutions are sequencing the genetic material from bacteria taken from nearly two hundred and fifty healthy people in order to unravel the relationship of our microbial "self" to our health, and they are seeking to perfect tools that will allow them to evaluate significant findings. There are many similar institutional efforts, but this federal HMP is the largest, best funded, and most coherent.

The first phase, which ended in 2012, sought to characterize the diversity and genetics of microbial life hiding within the nasal passages, oral cavity, skin, gastrointestinal tract, and urogenital tract. The current phase peers at human groups to collect data detailing both the microbiome's biological properties and microbiome-associated disease.[47]

Genome technology has provided tools that allow researchers to obtain DNA directly from samples and sequence it. For instance, the HMP is cataloging these bacteria indirectly by searching for DNA with 16S rRNA, a gene that serves as a bacterial marker. Thanks to these studies, we now know that by your third birthday, a delicate balance of environmental and developmental forces has cast your own distinctive microbial identity. Each person's microbiome is unique and each varies greatly, so two healthy people can have completely different microbiomes. And yet, knowing the composition of a person's gut allows scientists to profile the demographics of his mouth's microbes, although different organisms inhabit each site. Some researchers say they can determine whether a person was breast-fed; some even claim they can divine someone's probable education level from his microbial fingerprint, a statement that sounds rather...optimistic. Still, scientists hope all this will one day be useful in tailoring therapies to individuals.[48]

Although your microbiome will continue to change somewhat throughout your life in response to the same pressures that forged it—diet, stress, medications, age, and genetics—it remains as recognizable a biological signature as your blood type, for those who are able to read it.

Three bacterial groups rule our colons: Firmicutes, Bacteroidetes, and, to lesser extent, Proteobacteria. Fungi, protozoa, and viruses constitute minority populations.[49] Most human guts fall into one of three groups, or enterotypes, based on which bacteria is dominant. Enterotypes play a key role in disease susceptibility.

Jeroen Raes likens these enterotypes to forests. There are tropical forests, temperate forests, and bamboo forests. They're all forests, but they feature different species living together and functioning as a unit. He also points out that the environment of the gut is the food that you eat. People who eat high-fat diets have different microbial populations than those who eat more protein or those who eat mostly carbohydrates. That's important, he says, because more and more diseases are linked to a disturbance of gut flora—chronic diarrhea, obesity, irritable bowel syndrome (IBS), and, as you've read, "even autism, all have been associated with disturbed gut flora."

The connection is causal, not a mere association, says Raes. "Bad" gut flora actually cause disease. "If you take the flora of an obese mouse and you put it into a germ-free mouse, that germ-free mouse becomes obese....We're moving toward diagnosing people on the lifelong monitoring of your gut flora from feces."

Moreover, the environment these bacteria live in determines the variations in enterotypes, and the genetic signature of microbes helps explain why some people are susceptible to certain diseases while others enjoy immunity as well as why individuals react differently to various drugs and foods.[50]

Americans may find that overindulging in sushi carries dire gastronomic consequences. Japanese who live on a diet of seafood have evolved gut bacteria that can break down algae, apparently due to genes transferred from a marine bacterium called *Zobellia galactanivorans,* explains Ramnik Xavier. This allows them to digest sushi in quantities that those in the United States cannot, because the microbes are absent in North American populations.

Fat and Firmicutes

Speaking of food, rodent and human studies demonstrate the paradoxical role microbiomes play in obesity and overweight. The histrionics over the "obesity epidemic" are widely overstated; many fears promulgated by the weight-control industry and public-health leaders are not backed up by the facts. But there is no question that obesity is a serious medical issue in the United States, where more than one in three citizens are obese. That's 78.6 million people. The fact that Americans are growing fatter at younger ages raises the U.S. rate of metabolic syndrome, a connection between excess weight, insulin insensitivity, and high blood pressure that leads to diabetes, heart disease, and stroke— a dread trifecta. Obesity also encourages depression.

The *Diagnostic and Statistical Manual of Mental Disorders 5* pleads insufficient evidence to declare obesity a full-blown disorder. It speaks instead of binge-eating disorder, which, without purging,[51] "portends a greater risk of weight gain,"[52] leading in many cases to obesity. But anyone wondering whether obesity falls within the province of psychiatry need only attend an American Psychiatric Association meeting, as I did in New Orleans, and observe the wealth of workshops, panels, discussions, and lectures—to say nothing of the pharmaceutical advertisements—devoted to treating obesity. Or peruse the *American Journal of Psychiatry*, wherein obesity is discussed as a psychiatric condition requiring medication, counseling, and behavioral therapy in addition to bariatric surgery, candidates for which have a higher number of mental disorders than the general population. There is also research literature linking obesity to trauma; for example, to sexual abuse in young women. All this leaves little doubt that obesity falls within the purview of mental health.

But if we all live in the same country where cars replace walking, escalators replace steps, and commercials relentlessly tempt us with cheap, high-calorie, high-fat foods, why do only some of us become overweight or obese? An obvious answer is that some people eat better and exercise more than others. But this is unlikely to be the only answer, because in groups of people who have similar habits of eating and exercising, some still gain more weight than others. No one knows why.

Jeffrey Gordon and other researchers at the Washington University School of Medicine offered an answer when they discovered a large microbial contribution to obesity. Remember the three enterotypes mentioned earlier? One of them, Firmicutes, may be running the obesity show.

Some microbes, such as those in the clostridia and bacilli genera, are very efficient hoarders, extracting every bit of nutrition from foods. Moreover, these hoarder microbes also regulate gene function, encouraging their hosts to preserve more of this nutrition in fat. This helped our ancestors to survive when food was scarce and they had to work hard for each mouthful, but in today's world of drive-through triple-bacon cheeseburgers, ice cream trucks, and delivered pizzas, the hoarders' blessing has become a curse called obesity.

Gordon's team reported in *Nature* that the microbiomes of the obese, which differ from those of the lean, have especially high proportions of these hoarder microbes. When the researchers sequenced bacterial DNA from fecal samples, they found that the obese had a higher proportion of Firmicutes than did lean people.

So did fat mice. The types of Firmicutes in obese animals are more efficient at converting complex polysaccharides (carbohydrates that mammals need microbial help to digest) into simple sugars. Using this knowledge, Gordon took mice that had no microbiomes because they had been raised in a sterile environment and successfully manipulated their microbiomes to make them fatter or thinner by seeding their guts with microbes from either obese or lean mice.

Turning to humans, he put some overweight people on different diets and noted that regardless of whether the subjects were on low-fat or low-carbohydrate diets, their microbiomes shifted to the composition of slim people's as they lost weight. This would suggest that one's microbial population is a product of one's weight, not the other way around.

But another of his experiments, reported in the *Proceedings of the National Academy of Sciences*, adds a twist. When Gordon fed both the normal mice and the germ-free mice a high-fat, high-sugar diet, the normal mice gained weight, but the germ-free mice stayed lean.

The normal mice had microbes that, like a milder version of the hoarding microbes discussed above, made sugar more available to their bodies. And when researchers compared the two types of mice, they found that gut microbes in the normal mice regulated their hosts' metabolisms through two mechanisms. First, they suppressed *fasting-induced adipose factor*, a substance that encouraged mice to store fat. Second, they reduced the levels of the enzyme *adenosine monophosphate–activated protein kinase*, an enzyme that made it harder for mice to burn fat they already had. All this means that gut microbes release energy from food and encourage bodies to store that energy as fat while also making it difficult to get rid of the fat once it's stored.

Studies of obese people who undergo stomach stapling have found that their levels of Firmicutes change with weight loss, and their diabetes resolves too quickly to be attributed to the weight loss. Could microbes be responsible? Research is under way to find out.

Obesity is a complex problem born of both physical and psychological factors, and even within the ENS, many more factors are likely to emerge. Everything from genetics to childhood sexual abuse to the diet one's mother ate has been implicated, and the solution to the problem will not be as simple as going germ-free. But knowing that microbial balance plays a role enables us to look in a direction that could provide safer, more fruitful, and more permanent answers than the fat-busting pills of yore.

The measles, mumps, and rubella, or MMR, vaccine has been noisily demonized, leading distrustful groups and fearful parents to shun the vaccinations. Predictably, measles outbreaks have risen, and by late February 2015 a single outbreak that began at Disneyland sickened 123 children; most were unvaccinated. The first five months of 2014 saw more measles cases than comparable time periods in any year since 1994; the CDC reported that 90 percent of those cases were among people who hadn't been vaccinated.[53]

This rise in cases is a potential disaster, because measles is one of the most deadly and the most contagious of childhood diseases. In his landmark study of measles, Danish pathologist Peter Panum established this when he determined that of the 7,864 people living in the Faroe Islands in 1846, 6,100 of those who were exposed to the infection fell ill, an infection rate of 99.5 percent, and 23 of every 1,000 infected people died.[54]

Measles's carnage is not relegated to the past. In sub-Saharan Africa, measles still kills half a million children every year. But when I was a child and measles was ubiquitous, no one feared it. In spite of the deaths, pneumonia, and encephalitis it trailed, it was regarded as a mildly irritating rite of passage for mothers who had whining sick children underfoot. A familiar disease often breeds this sort of contempt, according to nineteenth-century Scottish health minister William Simpson, who noted the "peculiar fact, that the most dreaded diseases are the least fatal, and the least dreaded diseases are the most fatal...the disease that comes unexpectedly, and passes over quickly, is looked upon with greater feelings of terror than the disease which may be more fatal, but more common."[55]

If we need another reason to fear the measles virus, here it is: measles joins the growing number of microbes known to precipitate mental disease. Approximately one of every thousand children with measles develops encephalitis, a potentially dangerous irritation and swelling of the brain. There's also a severe long-term complication, subacute sclerosing panencephalitis (SSPE), a very rare fatal disease of the nervous system that occurs when children, usually younger than two, contract measles; their inability to produce certain proteins can allow the virus to survive indefinitely without evoking an immune response.[56]

Encephalitis symptoms appear within two weeks of infection; the disease kills 15 percent of affected children outright and leaves one in every four with permanent brain damage. SSPE symptoms begin months to years after the infection and lead to personality changes in the child—he or she becomes more irritable and argumentative and behaves erratically. Seizures and a stumbling gait follow, along with sensitivity to light and spastic movements, including involuntary jerking of the arms and legs. Cognitive skills begin to decline, resulting in memory loss, and the child becomes unable to walk. Speech is first impaired, then silenced. The child cannot swallow, goes blind, and is racked by seizures before falling into a final coma. Globally, only 5 percent of those with SSPE survive, but in the United States, lifelong treatment with interferon and inosine pranobex saves half of affected children.

In many cases of SSPE, the virus that is retrieved from the brain is abnormal and cannot be grown in culture. Scientists theorize that the virus mutated during the long years after the measles infection and before the viral destruction of the brain began.[57] Measles is not alone among childhood disorders in triggering mental illness; whooping cough causes ten times as many cases of brain damage.

Unfortunately, children whose cases of measles are routine and uncomplicated by encephalitis are not safe from mental disease. As many as ten years after they developed the skin rash, their personalities may begin to change, and irritability and erratic behavior signal a mental deterioration. How well they do depends on the particulars of their infection, but this scenario is not one that is considered by those who urge parents not to vaccinate their children.

The U.S. story is not the only one. Measles complications that threaten mental health are as common in the Middle East and regions of Asia as they are here, and there is no cure. The measles vaccine, however, has slashed the number of global cases.[58]

Fecal future?

We need to embrace novel therapies that don't involve decimating helpful bacteria or encouraging antibiotic resistance. Michael Pollan writes of one of these: "Fecal transplants, which involve installing a healthy person's microbiota into a sick person's gut, have been shown to effectively treat an antibiotic-resistant intestinal pathogen named *C. difficile,* which kills 14,000 Americans each year."[59] Today the transplants are done by colonoscopy or by a tube that runs through the nose into the stomach, but a 2014 study published in *JAMA* predicts that pills may soon be available, a more pleasant, safer, and cheaper technique.[60]

But as scientists decide which strategies to endorse, there is a further dimension of infection to consider that can dictate our collective, not just our individual, mental health. We must consider how the infinite variety of pathogens can distort the very nature of societies.

CHAPTER 5

Microbial Culture: Pathogens and the Shaping of Societies

No longer were there individual destinies; only a collective destiny, made of plague and emotions shared by all.

— ALBERT CAMUS, *THE PLAGUE*

Pathogens dictate more than individuals' mental health. There is a broader question to ponder: How do microbes influence people's tendencies to think and act en masse? Microbes shape culture in subtle but powerful ways, and they may trigger everything from exotic mental disorders that affect certain groups to genocide. Understanding the "microbial mind" may even illuminate predilections as subtle as our tastes in wine and perfume.

In 1989, an ophthalmologist approached the middle-aged Cambodian woman in his Long Beach waiting room. She sat silent and unsmiling as she gazed at the distant horizon. Her history read like the script of a horror film: somehow she had endured seeing her husband and son slashed to death in front of her by Pol Pot's minions, had survived months in a refugee camp, and had finally made her way, with her daughters, to asylum in the United States. Now she was blind, and she was not alone. At least a hundred and fifty women had presented to area ophthalmologists, and as Gretchen Van Boemel of the Doheny Eye Institute researched their cases, she discovered that they shared more than the same mysterious visual problems; they shared the same cruel story.

After seeing their husbands and children killed and being driven from their homes under threat of execution, these newly minted widows had walked hundreds of miles on infrequent morsels and gulps of water in order to save their remaining children's lives. Those who made it to the fabled safety of refugee camps found cold comfort in the sparse rations and lax security; rapes and muggings were common. Finally, the women reached the haven of America, but as the reality of widowhood, murdered children, isolation, and remembered rapes and assaults set in, a new blow staggered the women who had been torn from their cultures and left to eke out a lonely subsistence on welfare in a foreign land.

They were slipping into darkness.

Something was blinding the Khmer refugees, but ophthalmologists could find no physical reason for their sightlessness.

To professionals, this looked like textbook conversion disorder—the textbook being that of nineteenth-century neurologist Jean-Martin Charcot, who first proposed the conversion of intolerable memories into somatic symptoms that often have their origin in the person's culture. (Psychiatrists also speak of neodissociation, in which a person loses function but still processes stimuli—in this case, visual stimuli—that influence her behavior, although she is not consciously aware of it.)

Paralysis afflicts people who are conflicted about leaving home, and unexplained blindness strikes women who have witnessed a surfeit of horror. In addition, the slaughter of husbands, homelessness, violence, and exile effectively severed these Cambodian women from their traditional role in Khmer society in which a woman's sexual virtue, pleasant manner, and serene composure—traits embodied by the female deities immortalized on the temple walls of Angkor Wat—are integral to the family honor. A woman who is widowed, raped, degraded, starved, and driven from her home ceases, in a way, to be a Khmer woman.

Richard Mollica, a Boston psychiatrist who interviewed and studied these women, determined that after witnessing the horrors of genocide, they had willed themselves to become blind. They could bear to see nothing more, even through healthy eyes.

Yet as the women sat quietly in the waiting room, they showed none of the agitation one might expect in the wake of such trauma, now compounded by blindness and the unsettling absence of a clear diagnosis. A hallmark of conversion disorder is *la belle indifférence*, in which a patient shows an utter lack of concern about her state.[1]

Scientists are using neuroimaging, such as functional MRI (fMRI), magnetoencephalography (MEG), SPECT, and transcranial magnetic stimulation (TMS), to investigate, and recent research shows that specific patterns of brain activity are associated with conversion disorder.[2] One theory suggests that conversion is a protective strategy that derives from false body mapping caused by dysfunction in the brain's hypercomplex circuitry involving the cingulate cortex, insula, thalamus, brainstem nuclei, amygdala, ventromedial prefrontal centers, supplemental motor area, and other key structures. The primary sensory signals of vision, hearing, and touch pass through the thalamus on their way to the cortex, and these striatothalamocortical pathways constitute part of a feedback loop between the basal ganglia, which help govern motor control and motor learning. The motor plan starts in the cortex, is sent to the striatum of the basal ganglia, goes from there to the thalamus, and is relayed back to the cortex. Only then is it sent to the body, hence the cortico-striatothalamocortical pathway. Disruptions anywhere along this pathway, whether due to injury, infection, shock, or other psychosensory input, can cause false body mapping. The affected person loses access to senses such as vision or becomes unable to control parts of her body, as when a conflicted person becomes unable to walk.[3]

When such conversion symptoms grip many in schools, hospitals, army bases, or other closed communities, it is called mass hysteria.

On a brilliant fall day in October 2011, involuntary twitches and shudders suddenly seized Katie Krautwurst, a healthy, well-adjusted high-school cheerleader in Le Roy, New York. Doctors were baffled, especially when another girl soon exhibited the same symptoms, followed by ten more. By January, a total of nineteen teenage students and one thirty-seven-year-old woman in this small upstate New York town were at the mercy of frequent involuntary movements. These included spasmodic jerking, fainting, and Tourette's-like twitches and shouts. Many doctors, epidemiologists, and activists, among them Drew Pinsky, better known to TV audiences as Dr. Drew, and Erin Brockovich, descended on Le Roy, a working-class town approximately thirty miles southwest of Rochester. They sought to solve the case of the mysteriously afflicted Le Roy girls, as they were dubbed (despite the fact that a boy and a thirty-seven-year-old woman named Margery Fitzsimmons were also affected). Brockovich spearheaded a search for toxic chemicals, and Pinsky probed the girls' psyches while the cameras rolled, all to no avail.

An assortment of other epidemiologists and physicians proffered their own theories for newscasts and medical publications. In early 2012 the experts ruled out environmental factors, side effects from drugs and vaccines, trauma, and genetic factors. Pediatric neurologist Rosario Trifiletti from Ramsey, New Jersey, then stepped in to suggest that the tic-ridden individuals were suffering from PANDAS, explaining that infection with Group A streptococci might have caused the girls' bodies to produce antibodies that injured their nervous systems and led to the Tourette's-like symptoms. But as Susan Swedo pointed out, the girls' conditions did not really fit the PANDAS criteria. PANDAS is a rare disorder, which made it unlikely that so many would be affected within such a short time and such a limited geographical region. PANDAS is also unlikely to affect principally girls.

Undaunted, Trifiletti examined the girls and revealed on Dr. Drew's show that he had found evidence of strep or other PANDAS-associated infection in all nine of the girls he tested. Although he did not know if the levels of antibodies in their blood actually rose—a prime factor in determining disease—he declared that there was enough evidence to start them on antibiotics and anti-inflammatories.

In the end, Swedo was right: no evidence supported a PANDAS diagnosis. Instead, the Le Roy girls were diagnosed with conversion disorder, in which psychological stress causes patients to suffer real bodily symptoms. Epidemiologists concluded that the nation was looking at a case of mass hysteria.

How does psychological stress translate into bodily dysfunction? One theory indicts the amygdala, a region of the brain concerned with fear responses. It is overactive in patients who suffer from conversion disorder, Mark Hallett told the *New York Times:* "Ordinarily, the amygdala might create psychological distress, but instead, in these cases, it would create an involuntary movement." But Hallett, a senior investigator at the National Institute of Neurological Disorders and Stroke, added that while the theory was plausible, our knowledge of the mechanisms involved was still "primitive."[4]

Culture-bound?

Cambodia is far from the only country racked by displacement and genocide, but in the Khmer women, blindness in response to witnessing horrors is a culture-bound mental illness that shows why the insights of anthropology are as important as those of psychiatry in understanding mental disorders.

Culture-bound is the term psychiatrists and anthropologists use to describe mental disorders and syndromes whose expression is dependent on cultural factors.[5] Some are as dramatic as *koro*, a powerful panic attack engendered by the strong belief that one's genitalia are retreating into one's body. Affected women often believe that their breasts and genitalia are being reabsorbed, and all the afflicted believe that death will ensue. Possession by *koro*, not to be confused with the infectious kuru of New Guinea Highlanders, is often blamed on a malicious person who has stolen or shrunken the intimate body parts,[6] and the belief sometimes spreads, becoming a local obsession. Fifty-six accounts of genital shrinking or theft were reported in West Africa between January 1997 and October 2003, and news media recounted incidents in seven West African countries during 2012 and 2013. Genital-shrinkage anxiety haunts Asia, Europe, and even the United States. In China, it is explained as a reduction of the male yang principle; in West Africa, it is often laid to sorcery. This sounds absurd to contemporary Westerners, but the disorder has not always been a foreign concept; in medieval Europe, it was similarly believed that a man could have his male member stolen by witches.[7]

Other such disorders include amok, an episode of indiscriminate homicidal rage followed by amnesia of the event. Although it has been appropriated into English as the more benign phrase *running amok*, the disorder was first described in 1893 by W. Gilmore Ellis, British medical superintendent of the Government Asylum in Singapore, who observed it in Malays. Like *koro*, amok arises during times of social tension or impending disaster. *Pibloktoq*, or Arctic hysteria, was first described during Admiral Peary's visits to Greenland, and a disorder called *ataque de nervios* was documented by military psychiatrist

Fernández-Marina as the Puerto Rican syndrome, although it has been recently found among Hispanic peoples in the United States, including Mexican immigrants. Hsien Rin, a Chinese psychiatrist, first described *frigophobia*, an excessive fear of becoming cold, in 1975,[8] which was also ascribed to an imbalance in male/female elements.

Between 1890 and 1970, many other dramatic mental or behavioral disorders were observed among non-European peoples and classified as culture-bound.[9] These ailments were considered *exotic, unclassifiable*, or *unusual* by Western psychiatrists who did not always have a good understanding of the cultures they studied, and they labeled the disorders *culture-bound* because they differed from those in the European and North American patients they were used to treating.

Such ethnocentric classifications reflect the cultural myopia of psychopathology,[10] and *culture-bound* is an inaccurate term because it implies that the behavior occurs in only one culture. *Culture-related* is a better term, because many of these diseases appear throughout the world, even in the United States. *Ataque de nervios*—characterized by mental stress and symptoms of nervousness like decreased ability to concentrate, emotional distress, headaches, insomnia, gastric discomfort, vertigo-like sensations, and trembling—was described as a Mexican disorder, but it is found in many U.S. cities. How many cases of North American gun violence could be attributed to amok? Mental disorders appear in different guises in different cultures, and it has sometimes taken time, research, and a shedding of ethnocentrism to recognize this.

As a matter of fact, we in the United States and Europe have had our own seemingly culture-bound diagnoses: nineteenth-century vapors, or fainting spells; shell-shock, the symptoms of which change from war to war; and hysterical paralysis, which is an apt physical metaphor for the distress caused by sharply circumscribed women's roles. *Windigo psychosis* derives from a supernatural cannibal figure in Northern Algonquin mythology who can attack humans and transform them into cold-hearted cannibals. A Native American seized with fear that he is becoming a Windigo may fantasize about eating others while he is plagued with nausea and unable to tolerate normal food. This may progress to homicide or suicide.

Culture-related mental disorders are not limited to the exotica at which nineteenth-century Westerners marveled; today we recognize that they include variations of familiar diseases like schizophrenia. Far from being exotic and dangerous, the pathologies that Westerners label as culture-related disorders may help sufferers to better navigate life and society with a mental illness. As we shed Western biases in evaluating illnesses, it becomes clearer that culture-related diseases may disguise garden-variety anxiety or depression or the manifestation of illnesses such as schizophrenia, as in the case of *ataque de nervios.*[11]

Anthropologist Janis Jenkins has studied *nervios* among Mexican American families and observes that it is popularly used to describe a condition that would be diagnosed as schizophrenia in the West. In these cases, *nervios* softens the clinical picture of schizophrenia in ways that make it easier for the sick person to remain integrated in society and his family. Its recasting of symptoms also offers the mentally ill a less dire prognosis. *Nervios* is viewed as temporary; one may recover from it. It is also considered a disorder of sensitivity, overreaction, or an exaggerated startle response, not a psychotic derangement where people may be controlled by voices, unable to discern reality. Jenkins explains the important cultural function of this alternative diagnosis:

> Use of the term *nervios* affords a cultural protection not offered by other terms for mental illness, which are considerably more threatening. In their study of schizophrenia among Puerto Ricans, Rogler and Hollingshead (1965) reported that

both relatives and the afflicted individual go to great lengths to consider the problem as one of *nervios* rather than *locura* (craziness). As we have seen, Mexican-Americans also prefer the term *nervios*. This was particularly the case when relatives were offered a specific choice between use of this term and that of mental illness.[12]

Invoking *nervios,* Jenkins says, also helps cement family support by minimizing differences between the sick person and healthy family members. The term helps the patient as well, implying that his condition is temporary, whereas the words *schizophrenic* and *loco* connote a permanent, incurable state.[13] In this sense, says Jenkins, the culture-related diagnosis offers the schizophrenic a more benign social identity that eases their integration into families and society and has a better prognosis, creating the expectation of recovery. Similarly, a study of 1,031 rural African Americans, a population hit hard by the disease diabetes, found that the patients often referred to their condition as "sugar." Thirty-one percent of subjects who had answered yes when asked whether they had sugar later answered no to a survey question asking them whether they had diabetes. Subjects who believed they had sugar felt their condition was less serious than those who said they had diabetes.[14]

Anorexia, too, has long fallen under the rubric of a culture-related disorder. Until recently, it was perceived as a disease of middle- and upper-class WASP adolescent girls who, threatened by their incipient sexuality or a distorted body image, developed an obsession with being slim and avoided eating. A better understanding of how to recognize and approach anorexia is critically needed; its mortality rate is as high as 18 percent.[15] Anthropologists such as Caroline Giles Banks now recognize that anorexia is far more widespread than most of us think, affecting people from many cultures.

But, explains Banks, cultural rationales differ. In some

countries, anorectics are likely to refuse food more for religious reasons than cultural ones, which harks back to some medieval nuns who took pride in refusing to eat.

In other areas, anorexics report feeling too full or "bloated" to eat.[16] In fact, Banks described the cases of two American women from the Minneapolis–Saint Paul area who explained anorexia not in terms of the ideal of thinness but in religious idioms and symbols.[17] She reminds us that the United States itself contains many subcultures and that "anorexia nervosa's designation as a syndrome limited to Western cultures or to those cultures influenced by them may reflect unexamined assumptions on the part of researchers that dieting and secular ideals of slimness are primarily involved in the disorder."

What does this augur for the PANDAS/PANS theory of infectious anorexia? In cases of anorexia that seem to be founded in religious asceticism or some other cultural basis, can we rule out infection as the cause? As Banks points out, "While these symptoms are related in complex ways to biological dysfunctions caused by starvation and weight loss and may be, in part, unconsciously motivated... the anorectic consciously understands and gives meaning to her symptoms using culturally explicit and objective symbols, beliefs and language." So while GAS infection may be the physiological substrate for PANDAS anorexia, the affected person may impose a meaning on it that reflects her culture and belief systems.

Infectious mental diseases can also be culturally bound diseases, and anorexia is not the only example: kuru is an incurable disease of the human nervous system, often heralded by arm and leg pain, severe coordination issues, balance problems, difficulty walking, involuntary muscle spasms, tremors, and jerking. It causes rapid mental deterioration including emotional lability—the diseased person might, for example, succumb to deep depression that is abruptly supplanted by inappropriate and uncontrollable laughter. Dementia sets in, rendering the sufferer unable to speak or otherwise communicate, and people with kuru become placid and unresponsive to their surroundings.[18] Frequent headaches are common, as are swallowing difficulties that become so severe that the person is eventually unable to feed herself. It is a human analogue of the disease scrapie in sheep, and bovine spongiform encephalopathy, or mad cow disease, in cattle.

Kuru was first diagnosed among New Guinea's Fore people. Because men appropriated the pigs they hunted, the women and children supplemented their own diets by practicing a form of religious ritual cannibalism that involved eating the bodies, and especially the brains, of recently deceased loved ones.[19] Unfortunately, the prions that cause kuru are concentrated in the brain and nervous tissues, so 90 percent of the women in the area and children of both genders contracted the disease, but the adult men were largely spared. The Fore abandoned cannibalism in the 1960s, but the disease has a long incubation period, so as Robert Klitzman, director of Columbia University's Center for Bioethics, recalled during a 2015 telephone interview, "When I went back in 1997, cases were still appearing among men and women in their late thirties and forties." Kuru has been diagnosed as much as fifty years after the exposure to the pathogen.

Kuru has been regarded as a culture-related disease affecting the Fore people, despite the fact that quite similar prions cause Creutzfeldt-Jakob disease, or CJD, the clinically related disease that killed famed choreographer George Balanchine, as will be discussed in chapter 7. After years of illness, Balanchine died on April 30, 1983, and when his brain was autopsied, "chemical stains were added to some [slices of tissue] to help detect the pattern of appearance of certain brain cells and abnormalities, particularly the kuru plaques," reported Lawrence Altman in the *New York Times*.[20] Although Robert Sapolsky of Stanford University points out that the plaques of kuru and

CJD are different, this suggests that kuru is infectious despite the fact that it is culture-related.

Culture is important in determining not only which mental disorder exists but whether a mental illness exists at all, because behaviors can't be evaluated in a vacuum. A woman who eagerly feasts on human brains in the New Guinea Highlands of 1970 is participating in a ritual act that is meaningful and normal within her gender and culture. A woman who insists on ordering human brains at a SoHo McDonald's is likely to be regarded as having a mental disorder.

Genocide, an infectious madness

I've argued above that individuals suffer from mental disorders that may be both infectious and culture-related. But can societies suffer from such disorders as well? On July 9, 2011, the Republic of South Sudan emerged as the world's newest country, even as its government warred with armed ethnic groups within nine of its ten states. The armed clashes continue, hundreds have died, and tens of thousands of people have been displaced. In 2014, aid workers discovered fresh mass graves in this three-year-old country.

South Sudan has had plenty of company. Just in the past few decades, we've witnessed the Bosnian War of the early 1990s, Rwanda's 1994 ethnic genocide, and cars set afire by disaffected Parisians of African descent. Forty-five years after the Holocaust, neo-Nazi violence against immigrants soared in the wake of German reunification, and Germans have driven ethnic Turks from the country in droves. And the Middle East, of course, has long been synonymous with ethnic warfare.

Then there is the dizzying array of violent racial and ethnic attacks in the multiethnic U.S. "melting pot," from the slaughter of Native Americans to the kidnapping, torture, rape, murder, and violent revolts that characterized enslavement. This was followed by Italophobia, Hibernophobia (against the Irish), internment of U.S. citizens of Japanese origins, persistent anti-Semitism, racial segregation sanctioned by law, murders of rights workers, and burned churches and synagogues during the civil rights era and beyond. From the Ku Klux Klan to the Symbionese Liberation Army, the United States seems to have been intent on proving Black Panther H. Rap Brown's maxim: "Violence is as American as cherry pie."

In the struggle to understand the human penchant for racial and ethnic violence, academics have chased multifactorial social, political, and economic theories, few of which have helped stem ethnic and racial murder. Over the past half a century, some have even resorted to medical explanations. In the wake of racist civil rights–era murders, Harvard Medical School professor Alvin F. Poussaint suggested that the extreme racism that leads to murder and other acts of violence ought to be classified as a mental disorder. But American Psychiatric Association officials rejected his suggestion, arguing that U.S. racial and ethnic violence is so common that it constitutes normative behavior. The APA characterized even extreme racial violence as a "cultural problem," not a psychiatric one.[21]

"To continue perceiving extreme racism as normative and not pathologic is to lend it legitimacy," Poussaint wrote in response, adding:

> Clearly, anyone who scapegoats a whole group of people and seeks to eliminate them to resolve his or her internal conflicts meets criteria for a delusional disorder, a major psychiatric illness....Extreme racist delusions can also occur as a major symptom in other psychotic disorders, such as schizophrenia and bipolar disorder. Persons suffering delusions usually have serious social dysfunction that impairs their ability to work with others and maintain employment.[22]

The APA invoked culture as an alternative to psychiatry, but the two are not mutually exclusive; in fact, they are inextricably bound. In the biological sphere, *culture* refers to microbes coddled in an artificial medium where they are carefully tended under conditions favorable to growth. The broadest understanding of *culture* couldn't be farther from this definition: a society's shared beliefs and behavior—including their expression via symbols—that are pointedly *not* a result of biological inheritance. But both definitions are central to understanding how microbial culture has helped shape human cultures.

In the 1990s, gun-violence expert Dr. David Hemenway, a professor of the Harvard School of Public Health, determined that people living and working near gun owners begin to acquire, or at least to covet, guns themselves, and children of gun owners grow up to become gun owners, so that gun ownership spreads through a household and community in the same way the flu does, leaving debility in its wake.[23] A single gun eventually transforms a community into an armed neighborhood.[24] Hemenway's infection model of gun violence helps explain why the United States has more guns per capita than any other developed nation, and why nearly half of American men own firearms.

Hemenway has long clarified the vision of violence by following data without regard for conventional wisdom. His investigations revealed that a gun kept in the household "for protection" was forty-seven times more likely to kill an occupant of the home than an intruder. He found that whites are more likely to own guns than blacks, Republicans more likely to own them than Democrats, and conservatives most likely of all to own them. He found that the widely recommended gun-safety training programs for owners are associated with poorer storage habits; people who complete these classes are more likely than others to store their guns loaded and outside of lockable storage cabinets. And he found that most gun owners live in the suburbs and exurbs, not in cities.

The infection/contagion model sounds plausible because

we can easily see that those who live in violent environments become inured to it and prove likely to engage in aggression against others, especially outsiders. Whether these foreign elements consist of rival gang members, ATF agents, or members of hated religious or ethnic groups, violence becomes more common, as the APA suggested.

But Hemenway's thesis also echoes Poussaint's claim by conceptualizing violence as a sickness, something that infects and destroys a healthy community. A National Academies of Science study considers such violence pathologic and far from normal. Instead, it compares exposure to violence with exposure to HIV, tuberculosis, or cholera. Acts of violence are germs that target the mind rather than the intestines or lungs.

John Laub, a professor of criminology at Northeastern University, proposes a similar biological metaphor. Laub suggests that when children and young adults, whose still-developing brains possess great plasticity, repeatedly experience or witness violence, their neurologic functioning becomes deranged. He told the *New York Times* that "acts of violence lead to further acts of violence, creating a contagion effect and a sudden jump in crime rates that is hard to explain."[25]

A recent report that interrogated racial bias in U.S. imprisonment was headlined "Is Prison Contagious?"

Incarceration in the United States is frequently described as an epidemic, with per capita rates nearly quadrupling in the past 30 years. African-Americans appear to be particularly susceptible: In 2011, they were six times more likely than whites to be incarcerated, making up 38 percent of the 1.6 million Americans behind bars while accounting for only 13 percent of the U.S. population.[26]

Infection and contagion are not synonyms; infections are caused directly by agents such as bacteria, fungi, or viruses, and contagion refers to the spread of disease from one person to others by close proximity or touch. But some illnesses are both infectious and contagious. For example, the flu is caused by a virus and is spread to others through touch, coughing, and sneezing.

In 2012, a 153-page National Academies of Science report entitled *The Contagion of Violence*[27] summarized research describing similarities between the spread of violence and classic infectious-disease models. The report described acts of racially targeted violence as the germs that targeted not intestines or lungs, but the brain. It documented the tendency of violent acts to cluster, to spread predictably from one place to another, and to mutate from one kind to another, mimicking the spread of a viral or bacterial infection. Just as agents or vectors initiate a specific biological pathway leading to symptoms of disease, the report proposed possible mechanisms that govern the transmission of violence and suggested how the contagion might be interrupted. For example, one contributor, Gary Slutkin, told *Wired* journalist Brandon Keim that "the density maps of shootings in Kansas City or New York or Detroit look like cholera case maps from Bangladesh."

As the contagion model achieved critical mass, *Wired* asked, "Is It Time to Treat Violence Like a Contagious Disease?"[28] But this is the wrong question. Although scientists like Hemenway and Slutkin are proposing a *metaphor* of contagion, compelling recent research suggests that ethnic violence is not merely *like* a contagious disease. Instead, such aggression is the result of real physical, not metaphorical, infections or, more precisely, of our frenzied attempts to heuristically identify the signs of infection and thereby avoid them. We're not very good at it, and we end up with a lot of collateral damage.

Beyond mental disease

Microbes may shape not only frank disorders, but behaviors that are common to cultures. Whether we are xenophobes or xenophiles, belligerents or pacifists, conservatives or liberals, microbes are, as usual, pulling strings behind the scenes to help make us who we are. Evolutionary psychologist Mark Schaller suggests that microbes are responsible for what he has dubbed "protective prejudice," a suite of inborn thoughts and behaviors we have evolved in order to recognize and evade potential pathogens. Schaller, a professor of psychology at the University of British Columbia, calls this the "behavioral immune system."[29]

The regular immune system usually does a good job of routing invaders, he explains, but its efficiency in preventing disease is limited by the fact that by the time it acts, the microbial invaders have already breached our physical defenses, forcing us to expend energy and time neutralizing and evicting them. While we do so, sickness often prostrates us and even causes mental-health symptoms, however transitory. "If we can use our senses to detect infection risk—and then do something that prevents us from coming into contact with such threats—that holds tremendous advantages," says Schaller.

A 2010 study by social psychologist Chad R. Mortensen found that subjects who were shown images of sick people were quick to make "avoidant" arm movements in a computer game. They mimed pushing characters away, as if warding off a threat. Another study by his team at the Metropolitan State University of Denver revealed that participants who were shown discomforting images and given other information about infectious diseases rated themselves as less sociable than those in the control group did, essentially finding an excuse to avoid other people—and their germs. In yet another study, people shown illness-related images were more likely to express negative attitudes about foreigners. This unconscious avoidance reaction plays a driving role in ugly prejudices against anyone perceived as different, from those with different skin color to the obese to the disabled.

Worrying about parasitic infection correlates with anti-immigrant attitudes, and such biases are heightened at times when people feel more vulnerable to infection. For example, a study led by Carlos Navarrete of Michigan State University found that women tend to be more xenophobic during the first trimester of pregnancy, when the immune system is suppressed in order to protect the fetus from attack. By contrast, just after someone gets a flu shot, he or she feels protected from disease, and xenophobia decreases.

In an e-mail to the author, Robert Sapolsky noted that the literature also shows how "social conservatives are more concerned with personal hygiene, have lower thresholds for gag reflexes, and are more easily disgusted, than social progressives. And related to that, put people of all sorts of political stripes [in a room], have them fill out a questionnaire about various hot-button issues, and if there's a foul, smelly garbage can in the corner of the room, people become more socially conservative."

The legacy of protective prejudice is not all negative; according to evolutionary psychologist Ilan Shrira, author of "Guns, Germs, and Stealing: Exploring the Link Between Infectious Disease and Crime," "Pathogen threats strengthen in-group affiliation and solidarity (e.g., ethnocentrism, closeness to family), which creates a supportive network should someone in the group become sick."[30]

Steven Pinker's popular book *The Better Angels of Our Nature: Why Violence Has Declined* seeks to reassure us that mankind has enjoyed a dramatic reduction in violence over the ages. But even if he is right, the killing, rape, and torture of outsiders remains frighteningly common. This fact leads some scientists to ask whether humans might be biologically impelled to shun, drive off, or kill strangers or anyone who appears different. Such musings often hinge on political speculation or tortured data, and they typically involve some theory of a brain irrevocably hardwired by evolutionary forces to persecute outsiders.

This carries the whiff of something repugnant. The supposition that humans are immutably hardwired for xenophobia or frank racism implies that people cannot be held accountable for genocide or xenophobia, or, worse, that these are actual biological imperatives, not only beyond our control but also murkily sanctioned by the wisdom of evolution and the body; by "natural law."

Overreacting to a wide variety of strangers' germs and parasites seems at first glance adaptive, because the evolutionary price of infection by a pathogen against which you have no immunity is high. Just ask the millions of Native Americans who succumbed to European colonists' colds and syphilis, or the hundreds of thousands of nineteenth-century European soldiers who died of unfamiliar tropical diseases in the West African "White Man's Grave." Such diseases are bad for you, your community, and your future progeny, so your behavioral immune system decides "better safe than sorry" and impels you to avoid or eliminate strangers who might be carrying unfamiliar bugs.

But just as our species' humoral immune system frequently overreacts, triggering everything from hay fever to autoimmune disorders, our behavioral immune system also overreacts, attacking unfamiliar people who might be carrying dangerous pathogens. The body's evolutionary adaptations, and even evolution, often get it wrong and lead us to target groups and individuals who pose no threat.

The reason for such mistakes is that humans, unlike many other animals, are simply unequipped to distinguish infectious individuals from healthy ones with any degree of accuracy. Ants, Caribbean spiny lobsters, and bullfrog tadpoles can "sniff out" and avoid infected individuals that pose harm to their communities. Yale evolutionary biologist David Skelly has shown that healthy tadpoles appear able to smell chemicals associated with sick tadpoles. "When presented with an infected bullfrog tadpole," Skelly says, "the [healthy] tadpoles moved up to a foot away." Skelly went on to explain that many prey animals can change their behavior and even their body shapes when they smell predators nearby.[31] But humans have no built-in mechanism to differentiate infected people from well ones. Outside the laboratory, there are few reliable clues to pathogens, so we rely on indirect clues that suggest taint.

A person whose skin is riddled with pustules, bumps, or lesions may well be a victim of an infection, but we also tend to shun people whose skin is merely a different color than our own. It's true that people who travel to or hail from places where unfamiliar microbes live, whose sexual norms could change the sort or number of viruses they (and you) are exposed to, or who practice different kinds or levels of hygiene may be likely to harbor germs that you might acquire if you allow them to hang around. And conversely, they can acquire germs from you.

But in addition to fearing that giving strangers the benefit of the microbial doubt might prove deadly, we also bristle at outsider behaviors that often are wholly unrelated to infection. Speech, dress, foods, cooking methods, and even pets that mark outsiders are taken for shorthand that they might be pathogenic threats. According to the protective-prejudice theory, our fear of "the other" owes something to our fear of infection. Because we cannot accurately determine biological threats, the cost of xenophobia may well outweigh the speculative benefits of avoidance. Studies of countries racked by ethnic warfare provide strong evidence that using an infection model to describe ethnic violence is more than a metaphor. Xenophobia is an efficient incubator of genocide, says Randy Thornhill, who found that disease is the best predictor of ethnic violence rates worldwide, and a better predictor than poverty or income inequality. The more disease a country harbors, the more likely ethnic violence is. The official death toll of Rwanda's most recent ethnic genocide, in 1994, characterized by the mass slaughter of Tutsis by Hutus, hovers between 500,000 and 1,000,000, yet no biological difference between the groups that might pose an infectious threat has been found. The lowest estimated death toll in the 1992–1995 Bosnian War is 104,732. Both of the above figures include only those slaughtered outright, not those who disappeared or were raped, starved, or exiled.[32] "If you get high levels of xenophobia," says Thornhill, "then one group feels so negatively about another group that they want to kill them. So you get more large-scale violence like clan wars in regions with high parasite stress."[33]

Thornhill calls this phenomenon—which explains why some societies are more bellicose than others—a "parasite-stress theory of sociality." He theorizes that where harmful microbes abound, we find xenophobes who embrace ethnocentrism as a strategy for avoiding disease. Intergroup cooperation tends to increase resources, so ethnocentric cultures that erect barriers to intergroup cooperation greatly impoverish their environments, and that, in addition to the naturally impoverishing effects of disease, sabotages economic growth. To acquire needed resources, he says, "they are more likely to resort to violent conflict."[34] Global violence rates correlate with infection more strongly than any other variable.

The correlation holds true within the United States as well. A 2013 study by Ilan Shrira of Loyola University used data from the Federal Bureau of Investigation's 2009 Uniform Crime Reports to determine whether infection could be tied to changes in crime rates. Comparing that information with the Centers for Disease Control and Prevention's National Notifiable Diseases Surveillance System data revealed that rates of stranger homicide rise in areas with rising infection rates, but killings that target family members or acquaintances do not. Such correlations of stranger violence and infection do not prove that infection causes the violence, but they support the theory that a fear of the other leads to violent crime. "Under persistent disease threat," says Shrira, "xenophobia increases and people constrict social interactions to known in-group members. Though these responses reduce disease transmission, they can generate favorable crime conditions in two ways. First, xenophobia reduces inhibitions against harming and exploiting out-group members. Second, segregation into in-group factions erodes people's concern for the welfare of their community and weakens the collective ability to prevent crime."[35]

So we trade possible disease protection for certain community erosion, war, genocide, and wholesale death. However, despite our impulse to xenophobia, we remain the only species capable of using our intellect to understand and trump biological urges that we recognize as unfair or ultimately harmful. The human behavioral immune system operates on a higher cognitive level than that of any other species, and we should respect it.

But instead, we stick to our fallible prejudice-based method, as if preventing exposure to strange infections boils down to avoiding strangers or, more likely, driving them away. In fact, anyone whose behavior increases the odds of acquiring different microbes risks being ostracized, a fate that can be more deadly than we realize. Social psychologist Kipling D. Williams of Purdue University and his colleague Lisa Zadro found that, lacking resources and no longer enjoying the protection and social sustenance of their group, the shunned "lag behind, become decimated, and eventually die through malnutrition or from attack." In short, "Animals who are ostracized inevitably face an early death," and the same is true for people. "Although some humans ostracized by all groups have survived as hermits, the infrequency of such occurrences suggests that for humans also, ostracism threatens survival. And if not a threat to the individual, it is certainly a threat to the continuance of their genetic line." [36]

And we must keep in mind that for outsiders, shunning is at the benign end of the spectrum. In *The Nature of Prejudice*, Gordon Allport, a founding figure of the psychology of personality, describes a classic five-point scale of increasingly dangerous aggressions toward marginalized groups: verbal hostility, avoidance, active discrimination, physical attacks, and, finally, extermination via lynchings, massacres, and genocide, a progression that fits neatly within descriptions of delusional behavior.[37]

Fear, an infectious weapon

The fear of infection is a handy genocidal tool. Proselytizers of genocide are quick to inflame and floridly capitalize on such fears. The Third Reich's propaganda machine manipulated this fear of stranger infection, cloaking its racial hatred of Jews, Poles, and Afro-Germans in the language and imagery of infection. Such non-Aryans, Nazis claimed, threatened an (imaginary) natural order and so sabotaged the nation's purity and vigor. This purity was habitually couched in terms of biology, as when Rudolf Hess brayed in 1934 that "National Socialism is nothing but applied biology." More specifically, the Reich invoked the biological concept of infection to achieve *Gleichschaltung*, or "setting things in order." This was the "natural" biological order of things, to be achieved by cleansing the state of parasites, the inferior people accused of sapping the health, resources, and vigor of "true Germans."

One ominous image that adorned propaganda posters embodied the concept of *Krankheitserreger*, or pathogens, and depicted Jews, Communists, and gays as bacteria, symbolized by

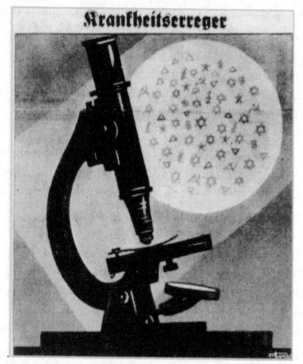

This National Socialist propaganda poster depicts Jews, homosexuals, and others as pathogens and threats to the health of German society.

small Stars of David, hammer-and-sickle icons, and pink triangles spotlighted in the field of a microscope. Polish Jews who had been forced into ghettos with inadequate space and hygienic services were decried as vectors of infection when the inevitable typhus and cholera epidemics set in:

> In the 1940 National Socialist propaganda film *Der Ewige Jude* (*The Eternal Jew*), rats teem while the voice-over reports that "where rats appear, they bring annihilation to the land... [rats] spread disease, plague, leprosy, typhus, cholera, dysentery, etc....just as Jews do among the people." Hitler not only referred to Jews as "bacilli" but also as "viruses" and "parasites," and he painted the Jewish population of the Soviet

Union as a *Pestherd* (plague focus). Heinrich Himmler, in a speech to SS officers in Pozna (then the German city of Posen) in 1943, made plain the equation of Jews with bacteria: "In the end," he declaimed, "as we exterminate the bacillus, we wouldn't want to become sick with it and die [ourselves]."[38]

A year after Hess equated Nazism with biological imperatives, Reichsbauernführer Richard Walther Darré declared, "As a Rhinelander, I demand: sterilization for all mulattoes with whom we were saddled by the black shame on the Rhine."[39] He was speaking of Somalian soldiers stationed in the Rhineland borders by France, many of whom had taken German wives and lovers. German Hereditary Health Courts judged the reproductive fitness of most persons on a case-by-case basis, but for black Germans and Afro-German children, visual or verbal evidence of African ancestry was enough to justify immediate secret sterilization in on-site clinics under Special Commission No. 3, which was established by Eugen Fischer in 1937. Frankfurt health office records for June 19, 1937, reveal a chilling example:

> The German citizen Josef Feck, born on 26 September 1920 and residing in Mainz is a descendant of the former colonial occupation troops (North Africa) and distinctly displays the corresponding anthropological characteristics. For that reason he is to be sterilized. His mother consents to the sterilization.[40]

Today the Stormfront site, run by an assortment of virulent racists who admire National Socialism, reproduces Hess's aphorism and screams "Expel the parasite!" as it makes its case for the extermination of African Americans.[41] In the 1994 Rwandan genocide, the Tutsis, like Jews in the 1930s, were dehumanized as cockroaches, rats, and vermin by those who were busily engaged in ethnic cleansing to "exterminate" them, another common strategy for identifying them as vectors of disease.[42]

Irish journalist Fergal Keane, who witnessed the 1994 genocide, wrote, "Tens of thousands became infected—and I can think of no other word that can describe the condition—by an anti-Tutsi psychosis."[43] Ibrahim Omer of California State University[44] determined that "genetic studies suggest that the Hutu and Tutsi of today are hardly distinguishable," but this finding has done nothing to dampen the demonizing so essential to genocide. Thus, protective prejudice, in its extremes, is far more than a historical concern, especially when it is deployed to stir up ethnic animosities.

Research by scientists like Thornhill reveals that microbes dictate more than crude impulses toward xenophobia and ethnic violence. Pathogens are also responsible for subtler aspects of culture, from social traits to politics. Research in the *Journal of Personality and Social Psychology* holds that in areas where disease is prevalent, people tend to be less extroverted.

The idea that extroversion and collectivism are national traits has prevailed for more than forty decades, bolstered by the work of Dutch social psychologist Geert Hofstede. In the 1970s, Hofstede investigated cultural differences in sixty-four countries that were home to national subsidiaries of IBM, where he once worked. To aid his research, Hofstede, now a professor emeritus at the University of Maastricht, devised a model of cultural dimension, a scale that measures, among other things, national characteristics of individualism or collectivism—in other words, whether people think of themselves as individuals primarily responsible for their own advancement, or as members of a social institution like a family, workplace, or society. Using this rubric, Thornhill found that nations that are heavily plagued by infectious disease, such as Colombia and Somalia, tend to favor collectivism over individualism. The United States has ranked highest in the world on the Hofstede scale for individualism, but within our culturally heterogeneous nation, collectivist areas stand out dramatically. Louisiana, South Carolina, and Alabama share high rates of infectious disease and a strong culture of collectivism marked by religiosity and an emphasis on clan ties. "You need a social network of reliable people in your group who will help you through the onslaught of disease," Thornhill told *Psychology Today* in explaining his findings. "That's the only health insurance that human evolutionary ancestors had."[45]

The individualism embraced by most citizens of the United States is not an inherently superior aspect of culture, nor is it better for mental health; in fact, nearly two decades of WHO studies argue that schizophrenics living in the collectivist nations of the developing world enjoy a better prognosis, which argues against the virtues of individualism, at least as regards schizophrenia. But collectivism *is* associated with the particular risk factor of infection-mediated violence. Afghanistan also has both high disease rates and a collectivist worldview marked by xenophobia and clannishness. It shares yet another social characteristic with similarly infectious areas: its people are *philopatric*, from the Greek words *philo* ("love") and *patra* ("country"), a term scientists use for animals, including humans, who do not leave their birthplace.

The apparent logic of preventive prejudice is hobbled by the fact that we cannot accurately determine infection threats; this means that the cost in genocide and warfare may eclipse the medical benefits of pathogen avoidance. Far from being slaves to our fear and disgust, we can apply reason to develop better ways of taming infectious threats, real and imagined, from strangers.

On an individual level, each of us can learn to overcome disgust, just as physicians and nurses quickly learn to do. We can learn to discard false fears of infection, as people did in the AIDS pandemic once they learned that while sex with an HIV-infected person without adequate precautions was risky, it was perfectly safe to work alongside, share a meal, or give a hug to someone with AIDS. Until these lessons were learned, the shunning, exile, "social death," job discrimination, and violence against the HIV-infected were open and frequent. In other words, the "hardwired" human biases are in fact as adaptable as microbes are, and as amenable to change. In addition, on a community or even a global level, the cost of prevention and treatment can be lower than the costs of wars, genocides, and bias-fueled violence. As disease rates plummet in response to this more reasoned approach to exposure risk, the rate of biases toward strangers should plummet too.

Not every microbial tweaking of human behavior and desires is pathological or weighty. Evidence is emerging that bacteria and viruses can fine-tune our appetites in a lighter vein as well.

Cat got your tongue?

There's no accounting for tastes, the cliché declares, but Stanford neuroscientist Patrick House might disagree. His work suggests that the subtle cultural influences of microbes may inform your tastes in wine, scent, and the gourmet Arabica in your coffee cup. Despite the self-congratulatory air of gustatory discussions that invoke *le goût friand* (and the heavy purse) of the gourmet, we may owe at least some of our refined tastes to a zoonotic infection.

What, for example, do Chanel No. 5, $350-a-pound coffee, and the elegant sauvignon blancs we crave have in common with jaywalkers, seductresses, and schizophrenics?

Not to put too fine a point on it: cat pee.

Consider that pricey java. Throughout the Indonesian archipelago, sharp-eyed promoters have underwritten extensive industrialized farming that capitalizes on an addiction once reserved for the very rich. Within endless rows of battery cages, Asian palm civet cats (*Paradoxurus hermaphroditus*), are force-fed one of their favorite foods, the coffee cherry. A day and a half later, workers reverently collect the "black gold" that these catlike marsupials deposit on trays installed beneath their cages. This culinary trophy is destined for the cups of the rich around the world.

Despite the aureate euphemism, this harvest looks exactly like what it is: pinkie-size logs of coffee beans bound by dark excrement. Once rinsed, aged, and roasted, these beans yield a gourmet brew that you won't find chalked up on any Starbucks menu. This is *kopi luwak* (the Indonesian words for "coffee" and "civet"), and it fetches $30 to $65 a cup, or as much as $350 a pound—about a quarter of the price of gold but as eagerly sought after.

Fool's gold, say some. Aficionados insist that the beans yield a brew that is "richer, sweeter, and smokier than any other bean in the world," thanks to their sojourn through the civet's digestive tract. This sublimity, they explain, results from the *luwak*'s discernment, as it selects only the finest coffee cherries, and also from the fermentation in its digestive apparatus, during which proteolytic enzymes free up amino acids that impart that irresistibly distinctive quality to the final brew.

But professional cuppers, those elite noses of the coffee world, often disagree. Many describe the taste as thin or nondescript and dismiss *kopi luwak* as gustatory bling driven by trend, not taste. A few critics add that the brew's quality has plummeted, pointing out that its superiority has long been ascribed to the free-roaming civet cat's talent for choosing only the finest coffee cherries for its dinner, while today's farms exercise no such discretion. Still other connoisseurs flatly dismiss the taste as tainted, moldy, and frankly fecal. In 1995, such professional skepticism earned *kopi* distributor J. Martinez and Company of Atlanta the loudest of critical raspberries, the Ig Nobel Prize.

All of which has done nothing to tame the cravings of devotees.

Moreover, snobbery alone can no longer explain the attraction, because *kopi* distributors now flirt with the mainstream. A down-to-earth marketer with thirty-three thousand likes on Facebook has promoted its wares to everyday folk, sans gourmet pretensions, as "cat's ass coffee." Its ads crow, "That's some good shit."[46] Now middle-class devotees join in the praise of the beans' alluring aroma as they acknowledge their *luwak* addictions. Taste, of course, relies heavily on scent, especially in aromatic fare like coffee.

These addictions may be more than metaphorical. What separates *kopi luwak* aficionados from its detractors may go beyond a slatternly palate and a slavish adherence to foodie fashion. Instead, an infection by the unicellular parasite *Toxoplasma gondii* may drive an irresistible attraction to the feline aroma in the beans.

The parasitology of desire

This book has presented the evidence for *T. gondii*'s causal ties to schizophrenia and suicide, but more than mental illness is laid at toxoplasma's door. A few hundred miles from the *kopi luwak* farms, Ajai Vyas of Nanyang Technological University in Singapore found evidence that toxoplasma manipulates its hosts sexually when it causes infected male rats to produce extra testosterone, enhancing their attractiveness to females. When they mate, males spread the parasite to their partners.

By increasing testosterone, toxoplasma also dampens fear responses, and infected rats may lose concern for their safety when they pick up the scent of a cat. At Stanford University, the group of Robert Sapolsky, professor of biology and neurology, found brain regions involving both fear responses and sexual attraction were transformed after exposure to cat odors and that, "somehow, this damn parasite knows how to make cat urine smell sexually arousing to rodents, and they go and check it out. Totally amazing."[47]

Although most of us long for escape upon entering a home that's redolent of felines, the power of *T. gondii* to make the scent of cat urine attractive may explain the appeal of *kopi luwak*: the 50 percent of the world's population that is already infected may be drawn to the feline scent in the beans. Although the high heat of roasting coffee beans should kill *T. gondii*, workers who sort and handle the roasted beans with ungloved hands and an indifferent approach to hygiene may ensure that the infection moves on to its previously uninfected human consumers.

And a connoisseur is born.

Some cat lovers go right to the source to revel in their pets' perfume, confessing on their websites that they cannot stop smelling their pets' fur. Some go so far as to specify the attractive scent of their cats' rear ends. Of course, only a small minority of cat owners seem to fall into the latter category. But why would anyone?

Czech scientists gave us a clue when they distributed towels imbued with the scents of various mammals, including cats, dogs, and horses, and then asked subjects to rate the smells for pleasantness. Most men who rated cat urine pleasant tested positive for toxoplasma. Just as the parasite evokes fatal attraction in an infected mouse, it can awaken irresistible desire in infected people because the same pathways and the same neurotransmitters, such as dopamine, govern the behavior of both humans and rodents.

The parasite transforms everyday behavior and, according to the research of Sapolsky and others, people's personalities. Once infected, the formerly cautious, light-averse mice swagger fearlessly into dangerous feline territory, and infected humans, even formerly cautious ones, tend to become thrill-seekers.

Unlike household rodents, First World urbanites have few

feline predators to fear, but they do face hazardous traffic, and for scientists, roadways provide the behavioral litmus test. Four large Czech and Turkish studies have found that the infected consistently take unnecessary chances on the road, both as pedestrians and behind the wheel. Infected drivers are two and a half times more likely than others to have traffic accidents.[48]

Eastern European researchers have found even more subtle personality changes: Infected men tend to be introverted and suspicious as well as oblivious to other people's opinions of them, which makes them indifferent dressers who are inclined to solitude. This would not seem to bode well for the parasite's future, as reticent loners are generally unlikely to engage in the sort of intimate social activities, like sex, that facilitate its spread. However, these men also have elevated testosterone levels, and women who are shown their photos rate them as more masculine than uninfected men. Why should this be so? Infection may well change the men's appearance because *T. gondii* affects their grooming behavior and their dress. For example, a man who stops shaving daily and sports stubble might be perceived as more masculine, male, or attractive. He may eschew his usual suit for more casual body-conscious gear like T-shirts or sweaters.

Decades of human studies also reveal a pronounced gender disparity. Unlike their male counterparts, infected women are *less* wary, more outgoing, and more interested in attracting others than are uninfected women. Coupled with the characteristic recklessness associated with toxoplasma, scientists theorize that these women are likely to be more sexually active than the norm.

Scent of a woman

Beneath the alluring apparel of the fashionable smolders perfume. No one has studied which scent *T. gondii*–infected women prefer, but ever since King Solomon imported civets from Africa in the tenth century BC, the ordure-like musk excreted from their perianal glands has provided an irresistibly discordant note to haute florals.

Although $2,000-a-liter civet musk is strongly repellent, minuscule quantities have bestowed a warm complexity to fragrances like Joy and Shalimar and to the rose, jasmine, and iris-root combination of Chanel No. 5 when used to stabilize the scents. Aphrodisiac claims are also common, although they are devoid of proof. Citing animal-cruelty concerns, Chanel stopped incorporating civet in 1998 and now opts to chemically reproduce the aroma in its laboratories, but the real thing remains a popular ingredient elsewhere. Some audacious perfumers even boast of rolling it about on their tongues in their quest to concoct a perfect scent.

Other renditions of civet are kinder to the palate. Sauvignon blanc is darkly complemented by a grace note of feline musk, this time in the form of 3-Mercapto-3-methylbutan-1-ol, or MMB, which arises as the grapes ferment. This chemical is the twin of a pheromone in cat urine, and this knowledge of the wine-and-pheromone kinship enhances rather than detracts from the wines' popularity, as new oenophilic monikers proudly proclaim the cat-pee connection.

On January 22, 2014, for example, Jessica Yadegaran evaluated Cat's Pee on a Gooseberry Bush, a 2008 New Zealand sauvignon, in the *San Jose Mercury News*. She proclaimed, "Cat themed wines have become a huge success, exceeding all sales expectations! It might not sound positive, but 'cat pee' is usually a favorable term used to describe the aromas in sauvignon blanc."

That same day, the *Week* enthused, "You'd think a Sauvignon Blanc characterized as smelling like cat pee would be awful. You'd be wrong." The unnamed author went on to note that it was doubtful that many had actually tasted cat pee; "they're really referring to a certain funky tanginess."[49] Neil Ellis Sincerely Sauvignon Blanc 2006, a South African wine, was heralded with "One recalls Sancerre and its characteristic gooseberry (often affectionately, or derisively, referred to as cat's pee). It is crisp and herbaceous, with mineral notes: a well-made wine that would be magic with salads."

No one has investigated the infection status of people who've made these sauvignon blancs "crazy popular," at least not yet, but my money is on their having the parasite.

CHAPTER 6

Winning at Evolutionary Chess: Strategies to Outwit Pathogens

The chessboard is the world, the pieces are the phenomena of the universe, the rules of the game are what we call the laws of nature, and the player on the other side is hidden from us.

— THOMAS HUXLEY

From its proud Viking roots and rustic cobblestoned streets to the chestnut trees shading verdant university paths, Lund is a southern Swedish town haunted, in the most charming way, by history. Fifty kilometers east of Copenhagen and about three hundred and fifty years old, the top-ranked Lund University is the oldest institution of higher education in Scandinavia. The centerpiece of its ornate campus is the restrained but opulent alabaster main building, its roof crowned with sphinxes.

But it was the university's starkly modern hospital of angled steel and glass that housed a contemporary life-or-death riddle that baffled Lund's ICU physicians: *ventilator-associated pneumonia,* or VAP.[1] In a 2010 *Scandinavian Journal of Infectious Diseases* report, doctors wrote of their attempts to address a longstanding worry: Patients on ventilators were developing pneumonia, a significant cause of death for critically ill patients who rely on these machines to breathe. Their lungs suffered invasion by harmful oral bacteria that they would not have aspirated were they able to breathe normally.

Sweden has no monopoly on VAP; it kills patients on ventilators everywhere. For those undergoing surgery that requires general anesthesia, who have lungs that do not function because of disease, or who are among the approximately 790,000 other U.S. residents[2] who need a machine to breathe, ventilators get oxygen into the lungs, remove waste carbon dioxide, and save lives.[3]

But in Lund, like everywhere else, doctors were running out of solutions for VAP.

The usual treatment was cleaning the mouth with antiseptics or antibiotics, which were also applied to the ventilator tubes. But doctors knew that relying on these tactics invited antibiotic resistance, as the bacteria evolved to thrive in spite of frequent applications, especially because the tubes were plagued by biofilms.

Bacteria in a biofilm stick together on a surface, like an oil slick atop water. Configuring themselves in this way allows bacteria to immediately glean orienting information about the number and position of cells in the colony. And why is this important? Consider a chessboard that suddenly materializes before a player who has no knowledge of the game in progress. There are things she'd need to assess quickly. How many pieces are left to her, and which ones—rook? Bishop? Knight? And what of her opponent's pieces? What does he have, and where are they located? For that matter, who is her opponent, and how skilled is he? Only when she has determined all this can she intelligently decide whether or not to proceed and with what strategy. She who moves without this information may reap disaster.

Bacteria in biofilms gather information about their relative positions using a murkily understood facility called *quorum sensing*, a collective sense of their own numbers and those of their neighbors of different species. As a result of what they determine, they differentiate accordingly, altering their behavior and organization toward aggressiveness or indolence. Complex, differentiated bacterial biofilms have an affinity for surfaces, such as ventilator tubes, that allow them to maintain their thin layers. As they form a slippery coat and adhere to solid surfaces, these microbial shape-shifters display an especially strong resistance to antimicrobial agents.

Bacteria that have developed resistance to one antibiotic often quickly gain resistance to others,[4] so by using another, Swedish physicians would merely be postponing the inevitable, and not for long. The doctors had to hit on a novel solution. They knew that resistance might leave them without a weapon against pathogenic bacteria and that truly frightening infections could proceed unchecked, causing many more pneumonia deaths. How, exactly, were the Swedish physicians to damp the growth of deadly bacteria while avoiding the specter of disease resistance?

Fighting fire with fire

Enter *Lactobacillus plantarum* 299, or Lp299 for short, bacteria that live in the mouths of most people and aid in digesting food. The investigators predicted that if smeared on the ventilator interface, Lp299 would successfully compete with pathogens for food and resources and crowd them out without causing disease. This plan was not perfect, because Lp299 could be aspirated by the patient and cause trouble in the lungs, just like the VAP bacteria, but the *Scandinavian Journal of Infectious Diseases* article mentioned above dismissed this hazard as a "calculated risk." Lp299, the doctors hypothesized, might knock out the pathogenic bacteria without the threat of antibiotic resistance.[5]

The scientists divided forty-four critically ill patients on ventilators into two groups. One group received the standard of care, which included cleaning their mouths and ventilator tubes with antiseptics, while the second group had their mouths and ventilator tubes coated with Lp299 instead. Investigators then looked for signs of VAP in both groups: they used chest imaging, watched for elevations in white blood cell counts, cultured their oral bacteria, and monitored the patients for telltale rises in temperature.

The results? "When we compared patients subjected to an Lp299-based oral care procedure with those who underwent the standard CHX-based oral treatment used at the department, we did not find any significant difference in the incidence of emerging, potentially pathogenic bacteria in the oropharynx or trachea." This small pilot study was reproduced in a larger trial that demonstrated that Lp299 was as effective as the commercial antiseptic in routing harmful bacteria that caused pneumonia—without the resistance hazard.

Using one microbe to fight another is just the sort of farsighted tactic we will have to perfect in order to shut down disease, including mind-altering infections, in the face of pathogens' ability to evade our medical strategies. Keeping up with microbial evolution is an unmatched battle, because while the average human reproduces several times during his or her lifetime, a microbe reproduces several times a day.[6] "Humans barely evolve quickly enough to adjust to rapidly evolving infectious agents," said evolutionary biologist Paul Ewald.[7] We are losing the evolutionary battle, and so we must rely on our wits to make up for our evolutionary sluggishness. We need to understand how microbes operate, stop making the same mistakes, and come up with more innovative strategies, such as the ones developed in Lund, if we are to have any hope of conquering infections and, specifically, infectious madness.

Futile tactics

At the dawn of the twentieth century, people frequently died from infections like tuberculosis and typhoid fever, illnesses that were a chief cause of infant mortality, which is the death of a child before his or her first birthday. The discovery of antibiotics allowed people to recover from bacterial diseases, and the medications did much more as well—they banished the surgical infections that made many procedures hazardous, assisted in cancer treatment, and, a few decades later, enabled the transplantation of organs.[8] As the significance of these magic bullets against disease became apparent, public-health experts confidently predicted the end of infectious disease,[9] and U.S. surgeon general William Stewart crowed in 1967, "The time has come to close the book on infectious diseases. We have basically wiped out infection in the United States."[10]

But as doctors used antibiotics profligately, microbes swiftly evolved to outwit them and change the game. This is in part because bacteria reproduce cleverly, supplementing their usual splitting with sexual reproduction to spread around the versatile wealth of genetic tools they needed to evade death by antibiotics. As antibiotic-resistant strains of bacteria evolved, scientists had to concoct more and broader-spectrum antibiotics. As if this were not challenge enough, more than a hundred new infectious diseases made an appearance in the decade after Stewart's display of hubris. Although one thousand antibiotics throng today's market, resistance has rendered many of them worthless, or nearly so. They cannot kill, or even neutralize, resistant strains.[11]

In 2013, the CDC calculated that two million Americans suffer antibiotic-resistant infections annually, and ninety thousand of them die,[12] more people than die from AIDS.[13] What's more, labs have not produced new antibiotics quickly enough to replace the useless ones. Nor are they likely to. Between 1980 and 2000, the FDA approved fifty new antibiotics a year, but from 2000 to 2010, only ten were produced annually. Since 2010, not a single antibiotic has replaced those rendered useless by resistance.[14] A 2008 European Centre for Disease Prevention and Control report calculated that only 15 antibiotics of the 167 under development had a novel mechanism.[15]

Antibiotic resistance affects the treatment of strains of anthrax, gonorrhea, Group B streptococcus, some forms of tuberculosis, typhoid fever, and methicillin-resistant *Staphylococcus aureus* (MRSA), but the overuse of antibiotics isn't just a product of concern for patients' health. Doctors are often pressured into prescribing antibiotics for viral disease, which the drugs will not affect. Seventy percent of the antibiotics given to animals are given not for medical illnesses but to increase growth and attractiveness. They are passed on in the meat we eat and in waste-based fertilizers, where they contribute heavily to the drug-resistance problems.[16] Antibiotics are added to soaps, over-the-counter creams, and foods such as shredded cheese.

Another prescient strategy for avoiding resistance is a back-to-the-future option called the bacteriophage. This is a virus that infects a bacterium and replicates within it, killing the microbe and releasing thousands of copies of itself in the process. It derives its name from *bacterium* and the Greek verb *phagein,* "to eat." A phage, as it is nicknamed, eats bacteria, and before the advent of antibiotics, phages were all we had to kill them.

Microbes are beating us at a game of evolutionary chess that our scientists didn't even realize was under way until the last few centuries—just a moment on the scale of evolutionary chronology. As if it were not enough that the pathogens within us outnumber us by trillions, they have also had an antediluvian head start. We've been playing as if the next move were all that mattered, racing to devise new antibiotics, then scrambling to replace them when the inevitable resistance saps their usefulness.

In 2011, researchers discovered that *T. gondii* deploys an ROP18 enzyme that neutralizes the ability of its hosts—including humans—to disable the parasite. We make proteins that erode the protective bubble in which the parasite cloaks itself, and toxoplasma finds a way to block the formation of those proteins,[17] another example of biological one-upmanship: the pathogen develops a defense and we disable it; we venture a chess move, and the pathogen counters it.

This game of chess has been going on a very long time, as we and our microbial adversaries have evolved together from the same early ancestors. Throughout humans' evolutionary timeline, we have been surrounded by what Paul Ewald calls a "coevolving cloud of colonists" in the form of pathogens and symbionts. As I argued in chapter 4, a simple "us vs. them" approach is nonsensical when our family trees suggest a parallel, overlapping evolution: Pathogens cause human epidemics, which are followed by our species' proliferation of defenses, including resistant genes. The disease rates fall in response, and the pathogen numbers nosedive to give way to a disease-free period, only to be followed by a microbial renaissance and more disease. This process tells us something important about outwitting pathogens and avoiding disease, including mental disease; it helps us better understand virulence.

Fierce creatures

Pathogens' broad repertoire of survival and propagation strategies depends on many factors. Ewald has pointed out how identifying the particular microbes responsible for specific mental disorders may help us to cure them. "We may one day distinguish between *influenza* schizophrenia and *T. gondii* schizophrenia," and treat and prevent them accordingly. We must learn to tailor treatments to the behavior and survival strategies of specific organisms, and that includes considering their virulence. And, suggests Ewald, microbial virulence is not that difficult to predict.

Knowing whether a pathogen is likely to simply annoy us with skin rashes, weaken and send us to bed temporarily, hobble us with paralysis, or kill us outright is essential. Among other things, knowing this tells us what sort of offensive is likely to work and what sort of medication side effects are tolerable; we'll accept greater risks and side effects to save our lives than we will to avoid a few weeks of fatigue and sniffles. Yet physicians have long treated pathogens as if all microbes behaved alike. Many assume, for example, that microbes necessarily lose virulence to become more benign over time, as smallpox, syphilis, and some other STDs have. And it is true that newly emerging pathogens like HIV or the Ebola virus, which have had very little time to evolve, are quite virulent. But virulence is just one move in the microbial repertoire.

Virulent strains thrive where the transmission is easiest. Consider three hypothetical strains of a pathogen: Impatience, which reproduces with alacrity and is quite virulent, quickly killing its host; Temperance, which reproduces at a moderate rate, causing periodic symptoms but allowing the patient to move about, go to work and the theater, and shed the virus during periods of wellness; and Indolence, so mild that the host feels well enough to go about his daily business and have a full social schedule every day but that sheds little virus.

Which strain will be the most successful? This depends on where they are. If the population is dense and crowded enough that the patient can infect many people in a household or community while simply lying in bed, Impatience will thrive. If the community of hosts is sparse enough that the person can spread the infection widely only if he is well enough to walk around, coughing, sneezing, perhaps kissing, and definitely spreading bacteria, Tolerance and Indolence will thrive, but Impatience will surge through a few individuals and die out when they do—unless it can find another way of getting around without human legs and breath. Microbes that can induce the correct behavior for the particular human environment will survive and reproduce, no matter their virulence level.

The late essayist Lewis Thomas was among those who argued that the most successful pathogens are those that keep their hosts alive, so pathogens evolve toward mildness and clemency. "Pathogenicity [the ability of a microbe to cause disease or serious harm] is not the rule," he wrote. "Indeed, it occurs so infrequently and involves such a relatively small number of species, considering the huge population of bacteria on the earth, that it has a freakish aspect."

This assumption of benignity is a common oversimplification. In sparsely populated locations like the desert or the Antarctic, a pathogen will find transmission difficult. When its hosts live miles apart, with relatively few social encounters, a virulent microbe will whip through a family or small social group and die out quickly without reproducing or spreading. Virulence is not necessarily in its best interests. Instead, "when the transmission of parasites depends on host mobility, natural selection favors milder parasites," Paul Ewald explains. "Take malaria. If we make houses and hospitals mosquito-proof, then we make it so that the only people who can be a source for mosquitoes are the people who are healthy enough to move around outside. So they're going to have milder strains, and we expect the pathogens that evolve to be mild."[18]

Thus, a microbe's virulence seals its fate when hosts are sparse—unless it is spread by a vector, a flea, tick, mosquito, or another wide-ranging delivery system, like water, that can transport it to the next host. Some virulent pathogens, like the blood-borne hepatitis C virus, or HCV, can survive for long periods outside a host; HCV lurking in the dried blood on razor blades or other surfaces can infect others months after an infected person has contaminated objects. Rather than making its way to the victim, a pathogen like HCV waits for its victims to come to it.[19]

Another strategy of a powerfully malicious microbe is to delay the onset of the illness so that the host can move around and spread the infection, as in herpes, which can be transmitted very effectively during the prodromal period, when an infected person does not yet have symptoms but is shedding the virus. Or it may not cause symptoms at all in some people, making them unaffected carriers who spread the infection. Mary Mallon, or Typhoid Mary, was an Irish cook accused of infecting dozens of people with *Salmonella typhi*, which causes typhoid. This happened during a period when Hibernophobia was rife, and Mallon was arrested and forcibly quarantined by public-health authorities at North Brother Island, where she remained for three decades, until her death in 1938. Mallon was unfairly singled out because, like polioviruses and hepatitis A, typhoid infects some people without making them ill. This allows them to circulate the microbes, infecting others.

But many microbes are not content to keep carriers well or passively wait for unwitting hosts. Instead, like the plasmodium parasites that cause malaria, they actively exploit the bodies and behaviors of their hosts for their own ends. The infected female *Anopheles* mosquitoes, which transmit malaria to humans, are significantly more attracted to human breath and odors than uninfected mosquitoes are.[20] Infected mosquitoes also bite more often and more aggressively. How does the parasite manage this?

When a noninfected mosquito drinks a blood meal, its abdomen stretches to accommodate it, sending signals to inform the brain that it has drunk its fill. The brain responds by ordering the biting frequency to abate. But in the infected mosquito, the malaria parasite intercepts the message, blocking the afferent signals in order to hide from the mosquito's brain the fact that it need not continue biting. The mosquito continues to feed, not for its own needs, but for its dark passenger's need to be propagated widely.[21]

Richard Dawkins calls such microbial manipulations an "extended phenotype"[22] because the genes of the pathogen are extended—expressed in the behavior of another animal; in this case, the mosquito. We don't think of malaria as inducing mental disease, but it does.[23] Depression is a common symptom

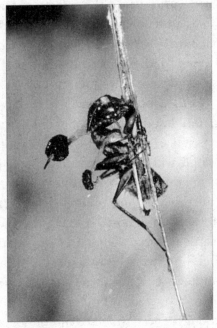

The idea that the one-celled parasite T. gondii *changes the behavior of rodents—and us—seems strange. But changing the behavior of a host to suit its own needs is a common stratagem of parasites. The* Cordyceps *fungus manipulates an ant in the Amazon into climbing a tree where the fungal spores can be more widely disseminated. The spore-bearing branches extend from the corpse of the ant.*

of the disease, but cerebral malaria also causes impaired thinking, memory loss, personality changes, and a tendency to violence. Soldiers who have served in areas where malaria is endemic, like Vietnam, often experience long-term effects that wreak havoc on their mental health. Nineteenth-century physicians reported the same long-term mental symptoms in returning English troops who had been stationed in India, and they recognized malaria as the cause. A 1998 study by the University of Iowa and the Veterans Affairs Medical Center suggested that malaria might be as significant a contributor to Vietnam veterans' mental-health problems as posttraumatic stress disorder and Agent Orange exposure.[24]

The same extended-phenotype concept characterizes the strategies of rabies, *T. gondii,* and *Toxocara canis*, a parasite that is carried by dogs and infects humans, blinding seventy people in the United States each year.

Rabies propagates itself by modifying its host's brain to exhibit murderously aggressive behavior. As it whips its host into an aggressive fury, it simultaneously courses into the salivary glands so that the virus can be spread widely. As noted in chapter 3, *T. gondii* invests mice, and us, with the boldness to swagger into danger, be it cat territory or oncoming traffic, and *Toxocara* does the same to us and our dogs.

For our safety as well as theirs, we must be wary of our interactions with animals other than cats and dogs. For example, the human penchant for delving ever more deeply into other animals' habitats, from the rain forest to the Antarctic, means that people often acquire infectious diseases from them, against some of which, like HIV, we have no defense. More are sure to emerge.

Some important infectious diseases, like cholera, typhoid fever, smallpox, rubella, pertussis, syphilis, and gonorrhea, are normally confined to humans, but many others are zoonoses, transmitted to us by animals. Besides the mind-altering toxoplasmosis acquired from cats and the *Toxocara* infections we pick up from our canine best friends, these include rabies, trichinosis, hantavirus, worms, and brucellosis.

Some pathogens specialize in attacking just one type of cell, as when polio infects anterior horn cells (the front gray matter of the spinal cord), and rabies viruses target neurons of the central nervous system. But other pathogens, like *Mycobacterium tuberculosis*, are *pantropic*, capable of infecting not only the lungs but many other sites, including the bones, skin, genitourinary tract, and the meninges (the covering of the brain), sowing confusion, lethargy, and altered mental status.

Although attention has been focused on novel infections like HIV and Ebola, and rightfully so, many other new infectious diseases result from an expansion of a pathogen's territory, expansions that we humans do much to bring about. Moreover, we are not the only species imperiled by our failure to give animals and their microbes a wider berth. Our pet dogs are infected with morbillivirus, the cause of distemper, which has killed unknown numbers of seals and porpoises around the world when undertreated canine wastes are dumped into waters. In the same way, *T. gondii* has expanded its habitat to infect marine mammals, even in Arctic regions, thanks to the same lax waste-dumping habits, which have also transformed marine ecosystems and opened the door to new pathogen infections.[25]

Virulent pathogens thrive when they can get around without us. "Sickness behavior" encompasses sadness, fatigue, sleepiness, lethargy. It is a strategy our bodies adopt when we fall prey to many infectious diseases, including some mental ones, like depression. It benefits the sick person to take to his bed, where he can conserve energy, aiding his immune system's battle with the microbe, and stay safe from predators in his weakened state.

But because sickness behavior consigns one to bed, too fatigued and sad to walk around spreading pathogens, the infectious organism that induces the illness needs another means of transportation. Cholera has found a solution: water. It prostrates its victims, but it also produces diarrhea, and the befouled water circulates *Vibrio cholerae* with terrible efficiency. Fleas infected with the *Yersinia pestis* hitched a ride on rats to carry the Black Death throughout Europe. Flea-infested rats also contributed to the 1918 Spanish flu pandemic, which was marked by mental diseases from neurasthenia to von Economo's encephalitis (also known as encephalitis lethargica), an infection that destroyed the minds of many survivors.

Virulence also changes with time and circumstances. "High pathogenicity and mutualism span an unbroken continuum along which organisms may move dynamically over evolutionary time," Ewald writes. Sexually transmitted diseases have often emerged with deadly virulence but co-evolved with us to finally show almost no signs of their presence. The ghastly running sores of fifteenth-century syphilis have yielded to a disease that is now nearly silent, especially in women. Today, gonorrhea and chlamydia also frequently lack noticeable symptoms.

This muting of symptoms is a cagey move by the microbe, because its chance of spreading during sexual activity increases if the infected person feels well enough for randy behavior and if her partner cannot see telltale genital eruptions that might otherwise give him pause.

In deciding how to counter microbial gambits, we must keep in mind that just as their relationship to us is not always black or white, pathology and virulence are not all-or-nothing phenomena. This ambiguity is illustrated by the bacterium *Salmonella typhimurium,* which actually repairs the damage it visits on its host. After breaking through the outer layer of skin in the intestines, this pathogen exudes a protein that helps to rebuild the shattered cytoskeleton.[26]

Evolving together, humans and their microbial guests have been playing such games for eons, but time is on their side.

Moreover, bacteria supplement their usual solo reproduction with sexual reproduction, which allows them to exchange genes, enriching their genetic diversity and their ability to evolve novel defenses. As a result of such pathogenic dexterity, genital herpes infects about forty-five million Americans, making it a very successful pathogen despite its low profile.[27]

Microbial faux pas

Our own missteps are as damning to us as microbial maneuvers. Officials contribute to viral propagation when they suggest flu shots rather than mandating them (for most); when they inadequately inspect food or store it poorly, which encourages the mental disease and limb loss of ergotism; and when they dump raw sewage, which efficiently transports pathogens, into the waters of the Global South.

Contrary to what one might expect, such blunders are not confined to the developing world. Despite Westerners' relative wealth and vigorous public-health infrasystems, they make the same mistakes, and more. I wrote of Third World waters, but the water of New York City is also home to an infinite variety of human enteric bacteria that can be found as far as a hundred and six miles from the city, thanks to years of dumping human waste. Poliovirus is among the pathogens found, a thousand meters deep, in the surrounding waters. For its part, Boston built pipes ten and a half miles long to ferry its effluents from the city and treated this sewage with chlorine for good measure, but some of the microbes in question are resistant to chlorine.

Other equally myopic tactics ensure that healing institutions teem with pathogens that can threaten minds as well as bodies. For example, the infected are herded into hospitals for state-of-the-art treatment, but this transforms hospitals into incubators of virulence. "Unfortunately, patients in a hospital are typically at a greater risk of infection than the general population due to medical conditions," warns a 2006 article titled "Infection Control in Hospitals."[28]

And no wonder. Concentrating many people who are infected, immunocompromised, or both in a small area provides a prime environment for pathogens to move from patient to patient with ease. And in easing transmission, as Ewald has explained, we encourage virulence. So it is not surprising that hospitals are the epicenter of so many especially harmful pathogens. According to the *New England Journal of Medicine*, "Between 5 and 10 percent of patients admitted to acute care hospitals acquire one or more infections, and the risks have steadily increased during recent decades. These adverse events affect approximately 2 million patients each year in the United States, result in some 90,000 deaths, and add an estimated $4.5 to $5.7 billion per year to the costs of patient care. Infection control is therefore a critical component of patient safety."[29]

Ironically, some of these failing strategies can be traced to human "success." Starting in the 1930s, during a giddy honeymoon with antibiotics, the medical establishment began to neglect important old-school protections, including physical barriers designed to stop infection transmission such as hospital rooms that isolate airborne microbes and use positive air pressure to ensure pathogens can't get out.[30] We should fully restore these infection-control designs.

Now the older infections such as tuberculosis have rebounded with a vengeance, and they are joined by newly emergent diseases such as AIDS, which causes a variety of mental disorders and suicide, and Legionnaires' disease. We need to introduce updated physical protections such as HEPA filters, positive- and negative-pressure rooms, and computer-assisted ventilation systems.

Even a hospital's layout affords an opportunity to minimize infection threats. Now that neonatal and perinatal influenza,

T. gondii, and bornavirus have been implicated in schizophrenia, it seems prudent to locate emergency departments and treatment rooms, which harbor a wide array of infectious microbes, far from areas where women deliver their babies and visit obstetricians, especially because future research may implicate other common perinatal infections in mental disease.

A report in the *Archives of General Psychiatry Research* about a Johns Hopkins Children's Center study found, for example, that pregnant women with evidence of herpes simplex type 2 infection gave birth to children who were nearly six times more likely to later develop schizophrenia.[31] Until the link is investigated more closely, it seems prudent to minimize pregnant women's contact with infections of *all* types, because pregnant women are dramatically immunocompromised during the first trimester to prevent rejection of the fetus. Laboratories housing dangerous infectious organisms abound in hospitals, and they, too, should be removed from areas near patient care.

The Semmelweis reflex

Danger also lurks in cherished badges of medical identity. In 2008, I often sat in the Seventy-Ninth Street Starbucks on New York's Upper East Side, and on any weekday, I could see a steady stream of harried health-care workers trooping through. Clad in surgical scrubs and white coats, they snagged caffeine fixes or lunch, their ties and stethoscopes dangling above a counter coated with the microbial witches' brew du jour, then flew back to the nearby hospital. As I watched them, I wondered which urban bugs were hitching a ride to patient floors on their ties, instruments, and lab coats. I noticed the same thing on New York's West Side, in Rochester, New York, and in Palo Alto.

Such seeming indifference to microbial contamination can

be found in the hospital too. Outside the operating room, necessary antibacterial vigilance sometimes proves a hard sell, as some physicians resist efforts to police staff hand-washing. Journals occasionally carry accounts of friction between surgeons and lower-status health-care workers whose job it is to monitor compliance with antiseptic technique. Despite a plethora of studies indicting medical vestments and tools in pathogen transport, too many caregivers are loath to surrender their microbe-bearing ties, white coats, and stethoscopes.[32]

I can't help reflecting on similar dynamics that frustrated Ignaz Semmelweis, a nineteenth-century Hungarian physician whose obsession with hand-washing was dismissed as an embodiment of superstition and old wives' tales. In Semmelweis's time, physicians and surgeons operated in street clothes with unwashed hands and lost one mother in three to puerperal infection, or childbed fever, which they unwittingly spread from one patient to the next. By contrast, midwives lost only one mother in nine. When Semmelweis insisted on hand-washing and sterilizing tools and surfaces with chlorinated lime at Vienna's General Hospital, he cut deaths to below one patient in a hundred. Yet his achievement became forbidden knowledge as he was roundly disparaged by other physicians. Some were offended by the implication that their unclean habits were killing patients, and all claimed that Semmelweis had no scientific basis for his protocols.

They were right. Because all this transpired years before Louis Pasteur demonstrated that killing microbes removed the threat of infection, Semmelweis could offer no logical reason why hand-washing and scrubbing reduced the incidence of fever. In the face of his medical marginalization, Semmelweis began writing ill-advised screeds decrying the "murderous" indifference of the medical establishment, and as a result, he was forced to leave his medical position. He was committed to an insane asylum in 1865, where he died after just seventeen days, only a few years before Pasteur validated his claims by popularizing the germ theory.[33]

Today, Semmelweis, venerated as a pioneer of antiseptic technique and a savior of women, is remembered for something else that has haunted many of the researchers featured in this book. The *Semmelweis reflex* is yet another name for the tendency to reflexively reject paradigm shifts, not because they are illogical, but because they offer new, discomfiting, and perhaps politically inconvenient explanations for disease. By now, this proclivity must be familiar to the reader.

No one questions the contemporary science supporting antiseptic technique. "Hand hygiene is probably the most important thing health-care workers can do to protect their patients from infection," says John Jernigan, director of the CDC's hospital-infection-prevention efforts. Yet, "despite years of efforts to educate both clinicians and patients, studies show hospital staff on average comply with hand-washing protocols, including cleansing with soap and water or alcohol-based gels, only about 50 percent of the time," reports the *Wall Street Journal.*

Public education and videos, some featuring Jernigan, urge patients to hold their doctors accountable by asking them to wash their hands. But how realistic is this? A June 2013 *American Journal of Infection Control* study found that "84 percent of patients were aware of infection risk, yet only 67 percent would remind a health-care worker to wash their hands, most often because of concern about appearing rude or undermining authority."[34]

In desperation, some hospitals, like the University of Kentucky Medical Center in Lexington, have resorted to linking merit increases to hand-washing compliance and even temporarily suspending the clinical privileges of doctors who ignore the rules.[35] This has worked.

But in yet another example of ill-conceived approaches to prevention, washing and disinfecting is often accomplished in the hospital with the ubiquitous antibacterial hand cleaners, even though soap and water banishes germs more efficiently. Physicians, who know better, often use the chemicals, which are not only less effective but also abet antibiotic resistance. Many include triclosan, an antibacterial blunt object that indiscriminately wipes out all bacteria. It even takes out those microbial communities that are necessary for health, like the anaerobic digesters used in sewage-treatment plants. These beneficial bacteria break organic waste down into small, manageable molecules such as carbon dioxide, methane, and ammonia. When we kill digesters with triclosan, we expose ourselves to harmful microbes in waste while simultaneously promoting resistant strains of dangerous bacteria.

The misplaced faith in the superiority of antibacterial chemicals over soap has led to triclosan's inclusion in toothpaste, dish soap, face washes, lip gloss, and even gym clothes,[36] all of which leach the chemical down the drain to impede waste disposal and encourage the very infections they are meant to quell over the long term. In the short term, they provide people with illusory peace of mind.[37]

Yet our health depends on our learning to curb pathogens and the mental disorders they cause with logic, not wishful thinking. This applies to some newer psychiatric medications such as selective serotonin reuptake inhibitors, or SSRIs, which are largely ineffective.

In 2010, a *Journal of the American Medical Association* study[38] found that a placebo worked just as well as antidepressants for the vast majority of depressed patients.[39] The University of Pennsylvania's Jay Fournier reviewed raw data from six well-conducted clinical trials and found that only the most severely depressed patients benefited from antidepressant SSRIs like Paxil and Prozac.[40]

People whose depression was mild, moderate, or even severe were as likely to be helped by a placebo as by their medication.

A flurry of other randomized, double-blind clinical trials—where patients are randomly assigned to get either drug or placebo and neither the patient nor the researchers know who is taking which—have validated this finding.[41] These antidepressants are among the most commonly prescribed drugs in the United States, and yet the results of the research done on them would surely astonish the one in ten Americans taking them.

In a few trials, antidepressants showed a quite small but statistically significant advantage over placebos. However, the term *statistically significant* is misleading. It refers not to the strength of the effect but to the likelihood that the results are real and have not arisen by chance. This does not mean that the clinical effect—how much of an impact the drugs have on mental health—is significant. In fact,[42] the evidence indicates that for most patients, the medications are worse than useless, because they are costly in both money and side effects, which can be life-threatening, especially for children.[43]

Given the antidepressants' price tags and side effects, the psychiatric community and the general public should not be satisfied with medications that provide only a marginal improvement over placebos.[44]

Despite this, the American Medical Association points out that antidepressant prescribing has not abated.[45] Readers, patients, and even researchers and doctors are often duped by unscrupulous advertising[46] and unable to judge the efficacy of psychiatric meds alone,[47] and the literature on SSRIs is particularly damning.[48]

But intriguingly, these drugs perform well in another role: they quell infection.[49] A 2012 study by Ross Tynan of Australia's Deakin University established that depression is linked with inflammation and that SSRIs and the related SNRI drugs greatly reduce inflammation of the microglia in the central nervous system.[50] In the journal *Brain, Behavior, and Immunity,*

Tynan looked at the ability of five SSRIs—fluoxetine, sertraline, paroxetine, fluvoxamine, and citalopram—as well as one SNRI, venlafaxine, to suppress this inflammation, and he found that they did so powerfully.[51] His study suggests that antidepressants may relieve depression and other symptoms of mental illness in a small minority of patients by muting the inflammation of infections that impair mental health.[52]

The failure of contemporary antidepressants to perform better than placebos undermines pharmaceutical-industry claims of, as psychiatrist Daniel Carlat puts it, "neurobiological wizardry" that allows the precise tailoring of medications to the chemical imbalances that are thought to produce specific mental illnesses. SSRIs are held out to counter depression by reversing falling serotonin levels in the brain, but if it is their antibiotic activity that discourages symptoms, this hints at the possibility of reverse causation; that is, falling serotonin levels in the brain might actually be a symptom, not the cause, of depression.[53] In *Unhinged: The Trouble with Psychiatry,* Carlat points out that the medications in each class of antidepressants are quite similar. The finding that these medications quell infection more effectively than they dispel mental-illness symptoms further strengthens the case for microbes' role in mental illness.

Prevention, with caveats

For all this chapter's focus on potential strategies against infectious illness, the savvy microbial chess master knows that prevention is better than treatment—especially for those infections that threaten mental health. "The most important thing, if you want to deal with mental disorders, is to prevent them from happening in the first place," Columbia University's Alan S. Brown told *Scientific American*.[54] The dwindling stores of medications are not the only reason why prevention is superior to drugs. For one thing, mental symptoms and diseases are among the side effects of many medications.

Doxycycline for malaria causes anxiety, depression, panic attacks, and hallucinations. Interferon for hepatitis C causes or worsens depression,[55] and HAART, or highly active antiretroviral therapy, drug regimens against AIDS, cause everything from paranoia, hallucinations, and persecutory delusions to catatonia, turning patients into mute, immobile "human statues."[56]

Even safe, effective treatments yield limited results, because little can be done to reverse infection-associated brain damage once the diagnosis is made. The slow fuse of infection that condemns many to schizophrenia, autism, depression, and dementia results from damage that has transpired over the preceding years or decades. Prevention preserves more brain function.

But we must be judicious in our choice of preventive moves.

For example, making flu shots mandatory, rather than simply suggesting them, could protect against the mental ailments the flu leaves in its wake, such as schizophrenia and von Economo's encephalitis. Even if this protection is incomplete, herd immunity could protect many fetuses from the subtle brain damage that can end in schizophrenia.

However, instead of mandating the influenza vaccine for all, the Centers for Disease Control and Prevention merely recommend that all pregnant women get flu shots. This may sound like a good preventive move, but it is precisely the wrong strategy, because it reflects a poor grasp of fetal risks. It is not an influenza infection contracted by the fetus that experts believe may cause schizophrenia down the line; rather, it's the friendly fire from the infected mother's immune response that harms the fetus. It is exactly this immune response that is triggered by the influenza vaccine, so pressuring all pregnant women to get flu shots will dramatically increase the number of fetuses at risk for schizophrenia. "I don't think they have considered this risk.

In fact, I know they haven't considered this risk," said Paul H. Patterson, the late author of *Infectious Behavior*. Thus, the best strategy to protect the next generation from schizophrenia may be to vaccinate everyone *except* pregnant women.[57]

Madness, worms, and friendly fire

At the age of twenty-four, *New York Post* reporter Susannah Cahalan was suddenly plagued by memory loss, delusions, a bedbug obsession, and crying fits that mystified her doctors. In her memoir *Brain on Fire: My Month of Madness,* she recounts how she was strolling through Times Square one evening when the lights became painfully bright, after which she emitted guttural grunts and her body was repeatedly racked by seizures. She became paranoid, convinced that her boyfriend was cheating on her. A battery of tests came up negative. She woke up in a hospital bed one month later, only the 217th person in the world to be diagnosed with anti-NMDA-receptor encephalitis.

It would seem, based on that statistic, that anti-NMDA-receptor encephalitis is a very rare disease—or perhaps it is accurate diagnoses of it that are rare. Patients who suffer from it arrive at hospitals displaying paranoid and otherwise delusional thinking, perceptual disturbances, agitation, changes in speech, memory loss, confusion, and agitated and bizarre behavior. They may also suffer involuntary movements, distorted consciousness, or even catatonic "statue-like" impairment of movement.[58] Unlike Cahalan, they do not always receive the correct diagnosis. Hers is an autoimmune disease; that is, it results from her immune system attacking her own brain and neural cells. Such autoimmune disorders can result not only from pathogens that get close enough to breach the immune system's defenses, but also, it seems, from keeping pathogens at bay.

Despite the clear need to put more distance between us and

the pathogens that can derange us, there's evidence that über-scrupulous hygiene carries risks too. The platitudinous "a little dirt is good for the soul" takes on new meaning when you consider the connection between the indiscriminate purging of microbes and mental disorders. When Louis Pasteur introduced society to germ theory and the microbial world's power to sicken, well-to-do Westerners developed a mania for mercilessly erasing their microbial neighbors. Unlike our eighteenth-century forebears, who bathed sporadically, whose hairdressers regularly cleared lice from their coiffures, and who shared their living quarters with rodents, we have lost our tolerance for vermin, food-borne parasites, and worms.

As microbial contact has fallen, rates of autoimmune disease, in which an immune system turns on its own tissues, have soared alarmingly, but only in countries where wealth and climate make a high standard of hygiene possible for most.

Malaise, fatigue, and other hallmarks of sickness behavior are common in autoimmune diseases such as multiple sclerosis, lupus, and rheumatoid arthritis. But a role for autoimmune dysfunction in psychiatric illness has been actively investigated since at least the 1930s, when autoantibodies were first reported in a schizophrenia patient. *Limbic encephalitides*, for example, include psychiatric manifestations as diverse as irritability, depression, hallucinations, and personality changes, with neurocognitive symptoms in the form of short-term memory loss, sleep disturbances, and seizures.[59]

In 1989, British epidemiologist David P. Strachan questioned whether the modern world's novel, historically unnatural reduced exposure to microbes could encourage disease, and as he amassed evidence that it was possible to be *too* clean, the hygiene hypothesis was born. Human immune defenses have evolved with their microbial neighbors closely for two and a half million years, so trying to get rid of them wholesale—friend as well as foe—may have been a serious blunder. Suddenly (in evolutionary time), the human immune system was forced to function in an alien, relatively sterile environment. Perhaps embracing a little more dirt can save us from diseases that threaten the body and mind.

Our microbial guests catalyze the maturation of our efficient immune systems, and so do multicellular parasites like worms, according to gastroenterologists Joel V. Weinstock and David Elliott. Elliott told the *New York Times* that worms are "likely to be the biggest player" in teaching the immune system to rout enemies. To test this theory, the duo fed worms to mice and found that this diet both prevented and reversed autoimmune disease. Moving on to human subjects, researchers determined that people with multiple sclerosis who were infected with whipworm had milder cases of the disease and fewer flare-ups. Whipworm infestation also improved inflammatory bowel disease, Crohn's disease, and ulcerative colitis. Each is frequently associated with psychiatric symptoms, often those of depression.

But other autoimmune diseases manifest primarily as mental illness. In anti-NMDA-receptor encephalitis, the disease that struck Susannah Cahalan, young women and children (and occasionally men) show sudden, mysterious behavioral changes that are followed by profound neurologic deterioration. The immune system makes antibodies that attack the brain's NMDA receptors, which are critical in learning and in the sophisticated mental functions that permit memory and multitasking. The victims suffer seizures, but they also experience a coarsening of their personalities, becoming paranoid and, in some cases, inappropriately sexual, depending on how extensive the area under attack is.

How could worm infestations possibly relieve the symptoms of this and of more common autoimmune diseases? Immunologists think a four-point response system of helper T cells—Th 1, Th 2, Th 17, and regulatory T cells—governs immune disease.

As Elliott explains, "A lot of inflammatory diseases—multiple sclerosis, Crohn's disease, ulcerative colitis, and asthma—are due to the activity of Th 17. If you infect mice with worms, Th 17 drops dramatically, and the activity of regulatory T cells is augmented." [60]

In 2008, John Fleming, a neurologist at the University of Wisconsin, decided to test whether consuming pig whipworms, which are harmless, could diminish MS symptoms in humans, and he put out a call for human volunteers. Jim Turk, a health-conscious athlete, master's student, and dad living in Madison, decided to answer the call and swallow 2,500 live whipworm eggs.

Jim had a good reason: "I was terrified."

After collapsing on the baseball field in the midst of coaching his son's team, Jim had been evaluated and diagnosed with multiple sclerosis. He knew that his body's immune system was stripping his neurons of the insulating layer that makes movement, thought, and sensory input possible. He also knew that if unchecked, this assault would eventually rob him of his stamina, energy, and, finally, his ability to move at all. He and four other subjects dutifully downed the salty elixir laced with worm eggs every two weeks, and at the end of four months Fleming found that of the average 6.6 lesions in each subject's central nervous system, just 2 remained. When the worm cocktails stopped, the lesions rebounded with a vengeance, to an average of 5.8. The fact that worms depressed the inflammatory response and the patients showed clinical improvement[61] is not ironclad proof, but it is quite promising, and Fleming is conducting larger trials.[62]

Naturally acquired worm infestations are far more common in the developing world than in the United States and Western Europe, a fact that may help to explain why autoimmune diseases show a pronounced geographic preference for the West.

Many wouldn't think of MS as a mental disorder, but in fact the disease affects the mind in several ways. Half of those with

MS have depression. Anxiety is also frequent, as are fatigue and sleep disorders, bipolar disorder, euphoria, pathological laughing and crying, psychosis, and personality changes. All these features of the disease provide "a complex interplay of biological, disease-related, behavioural and psychosocial factors [that] contribute to the pathophysiology of most of them," according to a 2010 paper in the *International Review of Psychiatry*.[63]

Mudhu's story illustrates lesser known psychiatric facets of the illness.[64]

Mudhu was late, but more than this was amiss. Her long black hair was oily and splayed unkempt about her shoulders; her blouse was smudged with dirt and had half-crescent perspiration stains at the armpits. Gone were the scarves, modest gold jewelry, and expensive shoes with which she'd once accessorized, and her body odor hung sharply in the humid air of summertime Kolkata.

Raised eyebrows and astonished whispers followed Mudhu to her laboratory bench. Hearing them, Ziba stole a backward glance and was alarmed to see that her former friend was standing rigidly before her autoclave, her eyes tightly closed. Her lips moved in silent agitation for a moment, and then Mudhu began muttering audibly to no one.

Suddenly her eyes flew open. Staring angrily at Ziba, she shouted, "Do you think I can't hear all of you whispering about me, trying to get me fired? Especially you, Ziba! Yes, I'm talking to you. You bitch! You are angry because we're both thirty but only I have found a husband, while you will die an old maid. I know you are blocking my transfer to my husband's lab because you can't stand the idea of our being happy together. You stab me in the back!" she shrieked. "You think I don't know that?" She emphasized her accusation with a rude hand gesture.

Mudhu was shouting so loudly that people had begun peering in from the corridor to see what was going on. Seemingly cowed, Mudhu turned her attention to assembling her instruments and fell silent. Tears stood in Ziba's eyes as she too returned to her work.

"I don't know what has happened," said Ziba at lunchtime to the technician across the table from her. "I've tried to talk to her, but Mudhu changed overnight after her marriage, barely returning my greetings, and speaks only of wanting to join her husband's lab. She seems to think there is a conspiracy to keep her from doing so and now…she is quite irrational on the subject."

More workplace outbursts followed, and her colleagues complained that Mudhu was unfocused, touchy, and full of wild accusations. They also worried because she often muttered to herself. She'd gotten married two months earlier, and since then she'd behaved very differently from the friendly coworker who had once gone out with them for drinks and occasionally brought in baked treats. Now she seemed to be mentally ill.

The quality of her work had plummeted alarmingly, and Mudhu's employer gave her a choice: Undergo mental-health treatment or be fired. In response to his prodding, she told Dr. Mukerji that she was extremely worried that her transfer to her husband's lab had been delayed due to "politics." After a few minutes, she accused her coworkers of a conspiracy to keep her and her husband separated, although there was no evidence that she was experiencing anything but the normal delay in transferring.

Neither Mudhu nor anyone in her family had ever been diagnosed with a psychiatric or neurologic disease. And yet her examination revealed a wealth of troubling symptoms that seemed to point to such an illness. These included an inability to concentrate, hearing voices, irritability, poor memory and reasoning, paranoia, poor hygiene, uncontrollable movements, the fact that she could not maintain rapport even with friends like Ziba, and delusions of persecution.

Was she suffering from psychosis due to stress? Dr. Mukerji

might have considered this possibility but for a telling sign: Mudhu's lips twisted downward when she smiled. He'd seen this before, and he ordered an MRI. The brain scan showed lesions in the temporal region that were suggestive of multiple sclerosis.[65] As it turned out, Mudhu was the one MS patient in one hundred whose first signs of the disease were psychiatric.

Next steps

Our tendency to overuse antibiotics has triggered both drug resistance and lasting damage to the microbial environment. Rather than churn out endless rounds of doomed antibiotics, we must embrace novel ways of quelling bacterial infections, such as those the dispensers of worm potions and the physicians of Lund have found.

The International Human Microbiome Consortium is one of the things we are doing right to control infectious threats to mental health. We must abandon our crude antimicrobial scorched-earth policies and use the detailed information about microbes we acquire from the U.S. Human Microbiome Project and elsewhere to craft evolutionarily savvy tactics.

Completely purging microbes such as the *H. pylori* that causes ulcers and stomach cancer is a shortsighted move that may condemn many of us to obesity, given what we've learned about the bacterium's protective role. The hygiene hypothesis warns that a failure to encounter some microbes within a still-unknown time frame may condemn a person to chronic illnesses like asthma and neuropsychiatric diseases like systemic lupus erythematosus, whose spectrum of psychiatric dysfunction includes cognitive changes, delirium, anxiety disorders, mood disorders, and psychosis.[66]

We should also revise our response to infectious disease based on facts we have long known but have relegated to forbidden-knowledge status. Lowering every fever, for example, undermines a key strategy for routing unwelcome microbes, which tend to operate only within a narrow temperature range. A fever is your body's attempt to turn up the heat in order to evict a pathogen; when you take an aspirin to lower the fever, you are laying out the welcome mat. In order to deepen our knowledge about microbial mayhem in the brain and block microbes' strategies, we must resist comforting mythologies, such as the assumption that pathogens always evolve toward benignity. We should also rethink medical practices such as the modern penchant for cesarean births, which are associated with abnormal microbial flora that may give rise to different health profiles and, possibly, to a concomitant rise in childhood mental disorders.

As Ewald notes, pathogens are far more virulent within hospitals than outside them, which suggests that doctors should look harder at any psychiatric symptoms that arise abruptly in hospitalized patients. Future avenues of research should include therapies that treat root causes instead of symptoms; address the mental-health vacuum of the developing world as well as the industrial West; and manipulate pathogen virulence,[67] just as *T. gondii* manipulates us.

Prevention is better than treatment, and nuanced measures such as exploiting herd immunity by mandating influenza vaccination for everyone except pregnant women and those planning to conceive[68] may prove sensible. If Laura Manuelidis of Yale is correct, some patients currently diagnosed with Alzheimer's or dementia actually have Creutzfeldt-Jakob disease, an infection caused by a prion. CJD is often avoidable by careful food preparation, just as we can steer clear of *T. gondii* by not eating tainted food and limiting contact with feline feces. CJD can also be transmitted by corneal transplantation, gonadotropin hormone therapy, and human-derived pituitary growth hormones, so we should develop a screen for the prion.

There's another possible answer: the future of infection control may lie with curators of bacteriophages, viruses that infect bacteria.

This unjustly neglected strategy is described in Anna Kuchment's 2011 book *The Forgotten Cure: The Past and Future of Phage Therapy*. Kuchment spins the romance of the discovery of phages in 1917 Paris by Felix d'Herelle and describes the decades of science and the violent politics of phage culture from Georgia to the United States. Stalin, for example, had the chief early proponent of phages executed, and the lives of both Tom Mix, the star of 282 silent Westerns, and Elizabeth Taylor were saved by phage treatment.

Phages have long been studied, produced, and used in Russia and Eastern Europe, cheaply and with great success, but we in the West abandoned their production when penicillin and other antibiotics promised to make infectious diseases obsolete. Now that so many antibiotics have been rendered useless by the evolution of bacterial and fungal resistance, we would do well to turn to them again. "We have to do something, because the old antibiotic approach is failing," Ry Young, director of the Center for Phage Technology at Texas A&M University, told *Popular Mechanics*.[69] "The problem is becoming worse, and becoming worse faster."

The advantages of phages are legion: Unlike common broad-spectrum antibiotics, the thousands of species of phages are very specific in their actions, each targeting one type of bacterium, so they do not trigger multiple resistance, nor do they harm the beneficial bacteria that we rely on to manufacture our vitamins and help us digest our food. This precision removes the danger of diarrhea, secondary infections, or leaky-gut complications, including autism, that sometimes ensue after a course of antibiotics. Phages are without toxic or harmful side effects, especially the highly purified medical preparations used to treat infection. In fact, we already ingest so many of them that

90 percent of our DNA belongs to phages within us that feast on the 90 percent of our cells that are bacterial—all without incident. This means that they can safely be used to combat bacterial contamination of food and may prevent infections in food animals more safely than the antibiotics we currently use. Moreover, phages are "smart" biologicals that reproduce and kill the targeted bacteria until no more remain, after which they are eliminated in excreta. Calculating correct dosages is unnecessary.[70]

It may not be long before we see phages on pharmacy shelves, because biotechnology start-ups are competing to produce phage therapy, which will give us another option against microbial infections that cause PANDAS, trypanosomiasis, and other mental illnesses.

Besides innovating such new ways of addressing bacterial infection, we must consider the needs of the poor and medically underserved who bear the brunt of infection. As mentioned earlier, diseases like general paresis are now found only among the medically orphaned of the Global South, and safe, effective medication for one of the most prevalent infectious mental diseases on the African continent has often gone undistributed,[71] as the next chapter will detail.

In short, our ability to reduce the incidence of schizophrenia, OCD, and other mental disorders tomorrow may depend upon the prescience of the moves we plot today.

CHAPTER 7

Tropical Madness: Infection and Neglect in the Developing World

The idea that some lives matter less is the root of all that's wrong with the world.

— Paul Farmer, MD, Cofounder of
Partners in Health

Acanit sat silent and unmoving on the bare and dented metal chair. It contrasted with her well-tailored knit suit, which Dr. Nabwire could not help thinking must be uncomfortably hot in the stifling air of the clinic's treatment room. Acanit's husband, Felix, had been gently bouncing their eight-month-old daughter, Dindi, on his lap, but he now stopped to complain, "My wife has been like this off and on for weeks. Now, she hardly speaks a word to me or our daughter. I don't know what she's thinking; she never acted this way before. Mentally, she has always been very strong; she is an exceptionally intelligent woman, but I don't know her anymore. What's wrong?" he demanded. As his voice rose in pitch and volume, he stared intently at Nabwire, as if he could divine the psychiatrist's thoughts.[1]

Acanit was an exceptionally intelligent and well-educated woman, a banker. She had been born and raised in Kampala, Uganda, then immigrated to Edinburgh. In her twenties, she went to London for graduate school. She met and married her husband there, and they'd returned to Uganda in the mid-1990s because he was active in national politics.

She'd adapted well to the quieter life in this small town until two months ago, when she became convinced that a knife-wielding man was following her. She began complaining that people entered their home in her absence and stole objects as varied as her financial documents, the baby carriage, and family photographs she displayed on the walls. She even distrusted the people in her church congregation and her mother-in-law; she said they were plotting to harm her. She refused all visitors, even her family.

She heard things. She woke her husband late at night to listen to the unbearably loud clicks that she insisted were meant to keep her from sleeping. She also saw things and people who were not there, and about a month before the visit to Dr. Nabwire, she started hearing the voice of God telling her that she was "anointed with holy blood." Around the same time, she began regarding her husband with suspicion. She said that she now recognized him as a servant of the devil, and she harassed him with prayers and loud warnings that their family could never be safe and complete if he did not repent.

The previous night he had come home to find her standing over their wailing daughter, shrieking Bible verses and looking at the child in a way that terrified him. Acanit insisted that she would never harm Dindi, but Felix decided to take an indefinite leave of absence from work so he could watch the child at all times, and he brought Acanit to his old friend Lutalo Nabwire, the psychiatrist at the HIV clinic.

Acanit was HIV positive, having contracted the virus in London from a former romantic partner. Felix was not positive and neither, fortunately, was Dindi; thanks to Acanit's HAART regimen of the drugs Combivir, nevirapine, and abacavir, Dindi was born HIV negative, and Acanit did not suffer from opportunis-

tic infections or other troublesome symptoms. Felix loved Acanit completely, but were he scrupulously honest with himself, he
would have had to admit that he'd brought her to this modest
HIV clinic rather than a large city hospital because he'd rather
have her treated where he could rely upon Nabwire's discretion;
in Kampala, there was always the danger of a scandal to be politically exploited. Now he'd begun to regret this. Her symptoms
surely had nothing to do with HIV, and she had no history of
psychiatric problems or any other medical problems. Nabwire
was an excellent doctor, Felix thought, but he should get Acanit
to a hospital with more resources.

Nabwire began to assess her mental state, and at first Acanit
was calm and fully oriented. She was aware of who she was,
where she was, and what day it was, and she insisted several
times, "But I feel well."

After a few minutes of this, she seemed to yield to fear and
anxiety and complained that she heard the clicking again. Soon,
she began shaking and shouted, "God has anointed me with
blood but the devil is interfering with me." She burst into laughter for a minute, and then fell into a stony silence.

Nabwire took Acanit's hand. "Why won't you speak?" he
pleaded. "I am trying to help you."

Then he sat back, deep in thought. He believed he understood what was wrong; he had seen this before. As he weighed
the words he would use to explain it to Felix, Acanit suddenly
seized Dindi and began to shake her while shrieking about God
and absolution of sin. It took both the doctor and her husband
to rescue the terrified infant from her mother's grip.

The nurse injected Acanit with a sedative while Nabwire
explained, "Your wife is having a bad reaction to the medicine
she is taking for her HIV, but don't worry. It is completely revers-
ible. We will keep her here for a while to treat her and find safer
medicines for her. Afterwards she will be fine."

"Do you promise?" Felix asked.

"Don't worry; she should be as good as new with a change of medicine," Nabwire assured him.

But privately Nabwire thought, *Yes, she will recover, but only because you can afford the new medicines she will need. They are expensive and becoming more so as supplies dry up. Few of my patients are so fortunate.*[2]

Acanit's story illustrates a troubling and often overlooked phenomenon. For a long time, I thought it was in the nature of bacteria to be democratic, infecting hosts without regard to station. However, this is not always so, and indeed we have engineered sources of bias that result in very different disease prevalences from region to region.

Infections that cause mental disease are especially devastating for residents of developing countries, in part because tropical and subtropical climates harbor many poorly understood pathogens and poorly medicated infectious diseases but also because the health-care vacuum and the studied indifference of many drugmakers separate people of the developing world from preventive efforts and treatments. This allows infectious diseases like malaria, polio, rubella, and general paresis that have been tamed or conquered elsewhere to thrive there. Of the seventy billion dollars spent annually on medical research, approximately 10 percent is devoted to diseases that cause 90 percent of the global health burden, leaving one billion people affected by undertreated tropical diseases.

The scope of these problems is sweeping enough to merit its own book; vast swaths of the Indian subcontinent, poor regions of the Americas, and even poor Eastern Europe enclaves suffer in a similar health-care vacuum, but because of sub-Saharan Africa's dramatic concentration of global disease, I will be focusing on examples from there to illustrate the issues.

Each year, up to three million deaths due to malaria and

close to five billion episodes of clinical illness meriting antimalarial therapy occur throughout the world, with Africa carrying more than 90 percent of this burden. Dengue, leishmaniasis, African trypanosomiasis (sleeping sickness), tuberculosis, malaria, HIV disease, diarrheal illnesses, and helminthic (worm) infections constitute some the most deadly infectious diseases. Children are the prime victims, as these infections sap their vigor, retard their physical and mental development, and, in many cases, shorten their lives.

Medical drought

Devastated by colonial rape, the depletion of its rich natural resources, and the dismantling and neglect of its original health-care institutions, much of sub-Saharan Africa has been left to poor health and a ravaged medical infrastructure, and few physicians remain. A mere 750,000 health workers care for the continent's 682 million people. The Organisation for Economic Co-operation and Development (OECD) estimates that this health-care force is as much as fifteen times smaller than in the thirty-four OECD countries that stimulate economic progress and world trade. Only 1.3 percent of the world's health workers practice in sub-Saharan Africa, but the region harbors fully 25 percent of the world's disease. This means that only one medical doctor practices in Africa for every one hundred in the United States, but the picture is even bleaker for psychiatric disorders: Nigeria, the continent's most populous country, has only one psychiatrist for every two hundred in America.

Worse, already sparse psychoactive medications are disappearing altogether as pharmaceutical firms abandon their development in favor of lifestyle medications for conditions such as erectile dysfunction and gastrointestinal distress. Moreover, new psychiatric drugs are expensive to produce, unlike the "copycat" medications, which are minor tweaks of existing pharmaceuticals. Because copycat drugs are cheaper and easier to make, drugmakers focus on producing them instead of concentrating on needed drugs to address neglected medical conditions.[3]

A European College of Neuropsychopharmacology report warns that retrenchment in the flailing pharmaceutical industry places "research in new treatments for brain disorders under threat" as corporate behemoths such as Roche, Pfizer, AstraZeneca, and GlaxoSmithKline eliminate teams, cut funding, and shutter divisions dedicated to psychiatric drugs.[4] The industry has been abandoning psychiatric medications since at least June 2011, when the *British Journal of Clinical Pharmacology* published an article entitled "Vanishing Clinical Psychopharmacology." That same week, David Nutt, a neuropsychopharmacologist at Imperial College London, told reporters that "these are dark days for brain science." At the 2011 meeting of the American Society for Clinical Pharmacology and Therapeutics, not one of the three hundred abstracts presented related to new psychopharmacological drugs.[5]

The wholesale abandonment of psychiatric drugs will be challenging enough for the affluent West, but it is disastrous for the undertreated people of the developing world, including vast swaths of Africa. This is because their access to these expensive medications is already woefully inadequate; any dearth will disproportionately affect the poor of the Global South.

In 2012, the journal *Science Translational Medicine* charged that the development of drugs for psychiatric disorders such as autism, schizophrenia, bipolar disorder, and depression has stalled as "major pharmaceutical companies recently announced substantial cutbacks or complete discontinuation of efforts to discover new drugs for psychiatric disorders."[6]

Although India has long been a source of cheap medications for the developing world, its role has been hampered by vigorous patent protection under the World Trade Organization's 1994 Trade-Related Aspects of Intellectual Property Rights, or TRIPS, statutes. A few developing nations, like Nigeria, manufacture many drugs, but 70 percent of them are generic, and the country engages in almost no new drug development.[7]

Western support is needed to supply psychiatric medication to the developing world. "Internationally, I believe the UN agencies like the WHO should be backing a global campaign," said John Kufuor, Ghana's former president and the special envoy for the Global Network for Neglected Tropical Diseases.[8]

In a perfect storm of psychiatric neglect, the dearth of psychiatrists and the scarcity of psychoactive medications has been joined by a wide-scale abandonment of antibiotic development. Profit-centered priorities of medical research have given us at least fourteen medications for erectile dysfunction but few new antibiotics and severely limited stores of the only fully effective medication against sleeping sickness, the most notable cause of infectious mental illness in Africa.[9]

"In recent years, the major pharmaceutical companies have been getting out of the antibacterial business," writes Deborah Gouge[10] as she explains that antibiotics are relatively unprofitable. Streptomycin and penicillin are seventy years old, which means they are off patent; this opens the door to generics and reduces prices. The short course of most antibiotics — less than two weeks — and the inevitable obsolescence caused by antibiotic resistance also limit profits. Of the thirty-six Western companies that made antibiotics in 1980, only seven remain.[11]

The lack of reliably available treatment for infectious diseases in the Global South will affect mental disorders directly, beginning with the challenges that deprived Africans of the only safe, effective medication against an epidemic killer and destroyer of minds. "When I think of infectious mental diseases," says Laura Manuelidis, professor of neuropathology at Yale, "I think first of sleeping sickness."

Sleeping sickness and mental havoc

As headlines blare news of AIDS, malaria, and Ebola, African sleeping sickness, or trypanosomiasis, seems to be forgotten, shrouded in silence. Yet sixty million West and Central Africans are at risk of contracting this parasitic disease, caused mostly by protozoa of the subspecies *Trypanosoma brucei gambiense* and transmitted by the tsetse fly. It resembles the familiar housefly, although the tsetse fly can grow to twice the common fly's length, and a long, beaklike proboscis sprouts from its head. Its wings fold with such precision that it often appears to have only one wing. But the tsetse fly is no mere buzzing annoyance. It delivers a prolonged, painful bite that deposits the trypanosomes that seal its victim's fate because they cause two regional forms of trypanosomiasis.

The disease is endemic to regions of sub-Saharan Africa and kills half of those it infects in the Central African regions of Uganda, the Democratic Republic of Congo, Sudan, Ethiopia, Malawi, and Tanzania.[12] According to WHO, during epidemic periods in certain areas, "Sleeping sickness was the first or second greatest cause of mortality in those communities, ahead of even HIV/AIDS."[13]

For months before their death, those stricken by African trypanosomiasis seem neither living nor dead, their zombie-like state brought about by the bite of the tsetse fly. The dying slip away exactly as they lived for the preceding year: silent, unmoving, and usually invisible. (A similar disease, American trypanosomiasis, or Chagas disease, threatens twenty-one South American countries, but it is caused by a different organism and requires different treatment.)[14] But before *T. brucei gambiense* kills its victims, doctors say, it drives them mad.

The fly's bite leaves a painful red chancre and is followed a few weeks later by the disease's first stage, known as the hemolymphatic phase, wherein the parasites reproduce in the victim's tissues, blood, and lymph fluid. The illness's early symptoms—joint pain, bouts of fever, headache, and itching for a few days—seem innocuous and are often ignored or mistaken for malaria because they resemble those of the malarial fevers that are common in affected areas. The parasite has to be detected in a blood sample or in lymph or cerebrospinal fluid to establish the diagnosis, but health-care workers are rare in the affected sub-Saharan areas, and so the disease often progresses unnoticed.

The body unsuccessfully tries to fight off the infection, and after several months the second stage ensues. It's known as the neurological phase, because the parasites, or trypanosomes, cross the blood-brain barrier to infect the central nervous system. The multiplying parasites cause the brain to swell, compressing blood vessels and evoking such dramatic mental signs and symptoms as behavioral changes, sensory disturbances, and a disruption of the circadian clock, coupled with confusion.[15] These produce an irresistible daytime drowsiness that is followed by nighttime insomnia.

We tend not to think of trypanosomiasis as a mental disorder, but we should, because the term *sleeping sickness* describes only its best known behavior change; the others are far more troubling. Cathy Hewison, an Australian doctor who has worked for Doctors Without Borders' sleeping sickness program in Sudan, explains, "It is an unpleasant and debilitating disease.... Symptoms include severe headaches and convulsions and people can become extremely aggressive and paranoid." Because of their aggressiveness, her patients often are strapped to their beds. A Doctors Without Borders report entitled "Saving Lives in the Name of Vanity" showed why when it described how, in

2001, one of Hewison's patients from Ibba village murdered his three-month-old niece while in a state of paranoid delusion. She adds that such events are not uncommon; a paranoid sleeping sickness patient once charged at her brandishing a plank he had torn from his bed because he thought she was trying to kill him.[16]

After six months to several years a victim may die,[17] but the intensity and prevalence of infections vary from region to region and even from village to village, wreaking the worst damage on children. The parasite can also be transmitted to infants through breast milk.

Within the past decade, at least three regional outbreaks have swept through Africa. Fifty thousand to seventy thousand people were infected in 2005 alone, according to WHO data. This is a very broad range, but the absence of public-health infrastructures in most of the affected areas makes precise disease surveillance impossible.[18]

The first stage can be treated with pentamidine, which is relatively safe. Or doctors can use suramin, at the cost of serious side effects. But most toxic of all is the traditional second-stage treatment, melarsoprol. This compound of arsenic and ethylene glycol, the latter of which is better known to us as antifreeze, is as toxic as it sounds, killing one person in five. Moreover, once the patient falls into a coma, melarsoprol is worthless, since it cannot cross the blood-brain barrier. In previous years, there was no drug that could arrest the disease once coma set in, and the infected expired on mats in darkened rooms or in forgotten corners of their untended farms. Although sleeping sickness is usually a rural disease, some died forgotten in the streets of thronged Third World cities.[19]

For decades, doctors could treat sleeping-sickness patients only with cures that seemed as dangerous as the disease and that could not help them once they fell into the final stage of trypano-somiasis. But hope arose in 1970 when Albert Sjoerdsma, former chief of Experimental Therapeutics at the National Heart Institute in Bethesda, Maryland, discovered eflornithine (also known as DL-α-difluoromethylornithine, or DFMO).[20]

Merrell Dow acquired the patent and set about testing eflornithine as a treatment for cancer and various illnesses. But in 1987 an announcement that Dow's new drug seemed to quell sleeping sickness threw long-standing economic tensions into sharp relief. In preliminary tests, eflornithine did more than simply relieve symptoms, like other sleeping-sickness medications; eflornithine seemed to be a true cure, killing the parasite by targeting an enzyme within it, ornithine decarboxylase.

The FDA approved eflornithine tests on human subjects in 1990, but the drug immediately hit a development roadblock: many pharmaceutical firms had a tacit prohibition against testing medications for use in tropical diseases, because those illnesses struck people without the means to pay high prices; there was no profit in it. Without such tests, the FDA would not approve the drug.

So instead, Merrell Dow continued to test eflornithine against cancer and other diseases for which a wealthy Western market existed. Fortunately, Simon Van Nieuwenhove, a Belgian physician working for the Belgian-Sudanese Sleeping Sickness Control Project, was able to obtain samples of eflornithine that he used on his own Sudanese patients.

The clinical tests showed eflornithine to be effective and safe, and it did indeed cure patients who had fallen into comas in the final stages of the disease, which no other medication had been able to do. Accordingly, researchers called it "the resurrection drug," and it was rechristened Ornidyl for use against trypanosomiasis.

But very few sub-Saharan Africans with sleeping sickness could afford Ornidyl's resurrection, and Aventis, which had acquired the patent, halted production in 1995,[21] citing its low earning potential.[22]

The firm began seeking other, profitable, uses for its drug. One was found, and Ornidyl was quietly reborn as Vaniqa, a fifty-dollar-a-month topical treatment for women's unwanted facial hair. Only after Doctors Without Borders discovered this and applied pressure to the drugmaker did it become available again for sleeping sickness, but not consistently so.

Let them take cake

As shocking as this withholding of medication from poor people of the developing world sounds, it is consonant with long-standing Western pharmaceutical policies. Of the 1,233 drugs licensed globally between 1975 and 1997, just four were devised to treat diseases of people in the tropics.[23] Little has changed since then. The drug-development-and-distribution efforts of NGOs like the Gates Foundation have been very successful, but they can help only a minority of people at risk for just a small sampling of tropical disorders.

One chilling change is that the industry's objections to providing medicines for non-Westerners are no longer tacit.

In 1996, Bernard Lemoine, director general of France's national pharmaceutical industry association, countered pleas that essential medications be sold to the developing world at affordable prices by saying, "I don't see why special effort should be demanded from the pharmaceutical industry. Nobody asks Renault to give cars to people who haven't got one." In January 2014, when India granted a compulsory license to ensure that Bayer's $69,000-a-year cancer medication Nexavar would be sold at a price that Indians could afford, Bayer chief executive officer Marijn Dekkers angrily called the compulsory license "essentially theft," insisting, "We did not develop this product for the Indian market, let's be honest. We developed this product for Western patients who can afford this product, quite honestly."

He is right that Indians cannot afford it, because the drug is priced at forty-one times the country's annual per capita income.

Thanks to this recent dearth of antibiotics and other medications, treatments for the Third World infectious diseases that trigger madness remain rare, expensive, and fraught with their own risks. Although some pharmaceutical firms now partner with the Gates Foundation and other NGOs to supply affordable medications, an excellent development, this does not meet needs. December 2014 reports gave some heartening news of reinvestment in anti-infectives by firms such as Tetraphase Pharmaceuticals and Merck, but there remains the question of whether these patent-protected medications will be available to the poor residents of the developing world.

Fortunately, there are some other routes to disease avoidance. Prevention in the form of vaccines, access to clean food and water, and even mosquito nets to discourage the transmission of malaria sometimes provide safer, cheaper ways to avoid illness, but as discussed in chapter 6, prevention requires careful strategies.

The secret strife of worms

In its medical vacuum, the developing world is plagued by diseases that are unknown or underexplored, so we know less about the endemic infections there that may trigger mental disorders.

We do know that rubella, which has been largely banished in the United States by vaccines (though it has recently mounted a comeback), is rampant throughout much of the developing world. According to Robert Yolken of Johns Hopkins, the rubella virus is on the short list of those thought to trigger schizophrenia when acquired in the womb or by the young.

Then there is the seemingly ubiquitous malaria. When the

238 • INFECTIOUS MADNESS

Plasmodium falciparum strain of malaria[24] attacks the brain, the result is cerebral malaria, characterized by progressive weakness, fever, coma, and brain swelling. It occurs in more than 575,000 people every year, most of them children younger than five living in sub-Saharan Africa. Without antimalarial treatment, it is always fatal, and even with treatment, it kills one in five of its victims. The survivors suffer a wide spectrum of neurological, behavioral, and mood disorders, from learning disabilities to blindness and epilepsy to behavioral changes so dramatic that they can be mistaken for schizophrenia.

This makes cerebral malaria a leading cause of childhood neurologic disability. Scientists still don't understand how the parasite that causes malaria damages the brain. Some believe that it causes the red blood cells it infects to pack tightly in small blood vessels in the brain, blocking them and disrupting brain function, but other researchers think that the parasite damages the brain more indirectly, through inflammation.

Even a newly discovered type of infectious agent, the prion, has been proven responsible for mental illness in the developing world. Daniel Carleton Gajdusek observed kuru (not to be confused with *koro*, which is discussed in chapter 5) among the Fore people in the New Guinea Highlands. The Fore called kuru the "laughing sickness" for its distinguishing facial muscle spasm, which resembles a malevolent smile — the same *risus sardonicus* that is an ominous sign of tetanus. Gajdusek claimed that kuru was contracted and spread by women who practiced ritual religious cannibalism. The infectious agents attacked their brains, eroding them and leaving them full of holes, or "spongy," hence the description of the disease as a spongiform encephalopathy. Gajdusek wrote that the kuru outbreaks stopped when cannibalism stopped, supporting his view that prions cause kuru. Robert Klitzman of Columbia and others confirmed Gajdusek's claims, but some of his scientific contemporaries contested them. They pointed out that cannibalism had ended in the community as far back as the 1960s and that the decline of kuru was concomitant with health initiatives such as placing hospitals, clinics, and clean running water near the affected communities.

The team Stanley B. Prusiner led identified the infective, self-replicating proteins that Prusiner dubbed prions in an attempt to capture their proteinaceous and infectious character. Like the endogenous retroviruses discussed in chapter 2, which resemble both genes and viruses, these prions occupy a twilight zone between two entities: protein and virus.

Prusiner, director of the Institute for Neurodegenerative Diseases at the University of California at San Francisco, met opposition from many scientists and writers who doubted that proteins would act in this manner. Some characterized Prusiner as a media huckster and gave his prion theory no credence. But he all but silenced them when he won the Nobel Prize in Physiology or Medicine in 1997 for his work. There are still those who remain unconvinced of the existence of prions, and perhaps the most prominent and accomplished of these is Laura Manuelidis, head of neuropathology in the department of surgery at Yale. She has published papers offering evidence that Creutzfeldt-Jakob disease might be caused by viruses or other well-established agents of infectious disease.

She also thinks it likely that CJD is more common than other scientists have assumed and that it may be causing many illnesses currently diagnosed as Alzheimer's.

Indeed, the case of George Balanchine, the Russian-born director of the New York City Ballet who is venerated as the father of American ballet, reminds us of how little we understand about CJD and its transmission.

Balanchine's symptoms first appeared in 1978; he began frequently losing his balance and falling while dancing, which forced him to explain rather than demonstrate what he wanted from his dancers. He complained that music sounded distorted to him and that color was so difficult to perceive that he had to abandon designing his own sets. Balanchine's balance, eyesight, and hearing gradually waned, and by 1982, he was incapacitated, as much by the mental confusion and memory loss he suffered as by the loss of control over his body. The man who had choreographed more than four hundred celebrated ballets "could not recall events that happened a few minutes before."[25]

The doctors who diagnosed his CJD after his 1983 death do not know how or where he contracted it, but in his *New York Times* column on Balanchine's diagnosis, Lawrence Altman mentions "a prominent neurosurgeon who had developed it, possibly from contact with a patient" and another patient who had developed Creutzfeldt-Jakob disease in 1974 after receiving a corneal transplant.[26]

In addition to familiar sources of infection like the plasmodia parasites that cause malaria and the unfamiliar prions behind kuru and CJD, there are many infectious agents of which we are unaware, especially in the health-care vacuum of the Third World, warns Robert Yolken of Johns Hopkins. He stresses that some of these unknown agents are likely to cause mental disorders.

However, physicians have long observed that even infestation with the familiar, ubiquitous worms and other parasites of the tropics can induce dire mental changes. Twenty years ago, J. Packman of Yale University wrote that "patients with parasitic loads are more likely to exhibit mental-status changes and there is an improvement in mental status of a subset of psychiatric patients following treatment for parasites."[27]

These risks have been quantified in other countries. German researchers studied thirteen hundred people with trichinosis, a disease caused by a common parasite people can acquire from improperly handled or undercooked pork. The initial symptoms include abdominal discomfort, nausea, diarrhea, vomiting, fatigue, and fever, followed by a second phase of muscle aches, itching, chills, joint pains, and seizures two to eight weeks after ingesting the tainted food.

It can also cause mental symptoms, including delirium, accompanied by insomnia and central nervous system inflammation, or encephalitis, which the Germans found in nearly one in four of their subjects.

Diagnosing trichinosis requires sophisticated analyses with antibody assays that were developed in 2003, and such technology is rarely available in the Global South. Animals infected with trichinella are "most commonly found in pork in the United States and Europe," according to the authors of *Psychiatric Aspects of Infectious Disease Syndromes* but this may not be so, because trichinosis may be dramatically underdiagnosed in the developing world.[28]

Neurocysticercosis is a common infection caused by a species of tapeworm in tropical countries. People in Latin America, Southeast Asia, and sub-Saharan Africa contract this from eating food contaminated with the eggs of the pork tapeworm *Taenia solium,* whose larvae accumulate in the victim's muscles, skin, eyes, and central nervous system, where they trigger epileptic seizures. The larvae invade the brain directly and form cysts that can be clearly seen on CT scans. The lesions and swelling they cause are also visible. Sixty-five percent of infected people also display mental symptoms, from depression to psychosis. Moreover, neurocysticercosis is the most common preventable cause of epilepsy, because 80 percent of the fifty million epileptics in the world live in the Global South, often in areas where *T. solium* is endemic.[29] Treatment requires years of the medications praziquantel and albendazole, which are not available in many affected areas. Fortunately, the preventive route can also help: handling and cooking pork properly and vaccinating the pigs that harbor the infection.

The disease was once rare in the United States, but it is

rising in incidence due to immigration, and WHO calls it the food-borne parasite "of greatest global concern." But control will be a challenge, in part because making a diagnosis requires a CT scan, which is rarely available in the affected poor rural areas.

It is harder to impute a mechanism to other infections whose signs are not visible, but the psychiatric literature is studded with documented associations between mental symptoms and parasites like giardia, roundworms, and *Borrelia burgdorferi* (the bacteria that causes Lyme disease), and these symptoms consistently vanish when the infection is routed, fulfilling one of Ian Lipkin's proof requirements.

Yet despite the wealth of infectious agents in the developing world, the dearth of medical professionals who can diagnose, or even suspect, any resulting psychiatric illness ensures that the diseases—and treatments—remain well below the public-health radar.[30]

The physical ravages of AIDS are all too well known, from cancers and a universe of opportunistic infections to wasting and debilitating symptoms such as oral infections and intractable diarrhea. But HIV destroys mental health as well. Few diseases wreak as much psychological havoc as undertreated HIV disease. The virus sabotages the central nervous system and brain, while the opportunistic infections it permits demonstrate the terrible versatility with which HIV promotes mental illness.

HIV is the most deadly infectious disease in human history. Thirty-five million people are infected, and seven of every ten of them live in sub-Saharan Africa. A UNAIDS report revealed that more than half of all people with HIV do not know they are infected, thanks in large part to the paucity of medical care in most of the developing world. In the West, the disease is largely controlled because people who are tested and learn their HIV status can benefit from effective treatment with highly active antiretroviral drug therapy, or HAART, sometimes referred to as active antiretroviral drug therapy, or ART.[31]

But in the developing world, such treatment is harder to come by. By late 2013, 11.7 million people in low- and middle-income countries were receiving ART, but according to WHO figures, this still leaves 22 million untreated people. This means that three of every five people in the Global South suffer from untreated HIV infection.[32] Fortunately, most—67 percent—pregnant women living with HIV in poorer countries do receive ART, which can prevent the transmission of HIV to their unborn children.

We know that people with HIV are more likely than uninfected people to suffer psychosis and commit suicide. Ninety percent of the people with HIV who experience psychosis fall prey to delusions that they are being persecuted or even that others are transmitting thoughts into their minds. Hallucinations (usually hearing voices) and confusion also occur. But they may also be subject to emotional states that veer from profound depression to irritation to euphoria. Experts estimate that as many as 40 percent of U.S. residents living with HIV suffer from anxiety disorders.[33]

However, experts still disagree on just how the virus drives mental illness. The psychosocial stress of having a chronic disease that impairs health, requires constant monitoring, and carries a social stigma certainly increases the risk of anxiety and other mental symptoms, but researchers believe that the virus itself also causes dementia and psychosis in approximately 15 percent of people with HIV.[34] The virus causes psychosis by various means, some of which interact.

AIDS dementia complex, or ADC,[35] leads to cognitive decline and lessens the ability to focus, think, concentrate, and problem solve.

A 2013 report in the *German Journal of Psychiatry* analyzed forty-seven studies of HIV and psychiatric disturbances published from 1970 to January 2012.[36] The authors found that the direct effects of the virus on the central nervous system could produce cancers and organic brain syndromes that included dementia and psychosis. To give just one example, the virus encourages free calcium to flood the spaces between cells, and calcium levels drive neurotransmitter release, so the finely coordinated firing of synapses in the brain becomes wildly inappropriate, disrupting interneuron communication and affecting a wide variety of brain functions.[37]

Such brain dysfunction usually appears in late-stage HIV infection, typically after the disease has progressed to full-blown AIDS, but most affected patients are still in their thirties. The mental disturbances, like the mechanisms HIV uses to assail the mind, are legion—paranoid delusions, hallucinations, cognitive impairment that prevents logical thought, memory loss. Less frequently, HIV causes catatonia resembling that suffered by survivors of the 1918 epidemic of encephalitis lethargica, or sleeping sickness, who were treated by Oliver Sacks as described in *Awakenings.*

But other factors also spur patients' mental derangement—opportunistic infections, the failure of a weakened immune system to fight off attacks on the brain by other pathogens like the tuberculosis bacterium or the *T. gondii* parasite, and the substance-abuse disorders found in disproportionate numbers of people with HIV. The German study also unveiled a terrible synergy in the ravages of HIV on mental health. People with HIV who develop psychosis suffer greater neurological impairment, and so do those who have a history of drug abuse. The infected with histories of drug abuse are also likely to fare more poorly and die earlier than other people with HIV and AIDS, leading the authors to conclude, "The high co-prevalence suggests a possible [causal] association between HIV infection and psychosis."[38]

The variety of HIV-related psychoses are treated by conventional antipsychotics, but fortunately, most people don't need them for long; the psychotic symptoms tend to abate as their physical disease is brought under control. This is a good thing, because even the medications used to treat HIV can contribute to dementia and psychosis. For example, up to half of those who take efavirenz as part of their drug therapy experience vivid dreams, nightmares, insomnia, and mood symptoms. These mild disturbances seem far outweighed by the medication's benefits, but others suffer more significant psychiatric problems, including mania, depression, suicidal thoughts, psychosis, and hallucinations.

Genetics also plays a role. Cytochrome P-450 is a major enzyme involved in drug metabolism, and those people with a particular variant of the gene that codes for it are more likely to respond to efavirenz with psychosis. This is an important risk factor for Ugandans as well as for Western Europeans; doctors should monitor patients on efavirenz closely, but this is less likely to happen in the developing world, where just getting HAART to HIV-positive people is a challenge.[39]

Hazards of modernity

In order to reduce HIV infections and other diseases, the UN mandates antenatal care in a health facility as part of the Millennium Development Goal (MDG), and various well-intentioned campaigns urge mothers-to-be to give birth in hospitals. Yet recent discoveries belie the assumption that giving birth at a hospital is always the best way for Africans to avoid infection.[40]

In the representative African countries of Kenya, Tanzania, and Zambia, wealthier, employed, better-educated, urban-dwelling women are more, not less, likely to be infected with HIV. These are also the women who are most likely to give birth in a hospital. Part of the problem, as I discussed in a 2007 *New*

York Times editorial, is the spread of HIV by well-meaning health-care workers struggling to give quality care under deplorable conditions that often preclude effective infection control.

Meticulous sterile technique is needed to prevent the spread of HIV, trypanosomiasis, and other diseases that can imperil mental health. But in poor undeveloped countries, safe devices are as scarce as doctors. Despite an unsupported assumption that the AIDS crisis in Africa is mostly fueled by patient careless-ness and sexual promiscuity, reused SUDs (single-use devices) and unsterilized needles help to spread infectious illnesses throughout Africa with terrible efficiency. *POZ* blogger Simon Collery wrote,

> It is not known what proportion of HIV transmission is a result of sexual intercourse and what proportion is a result of other modes of transmission, such as exposure to contami-nated medical instruments, unsafe cosmetic or traditional practices.... The assumption that most transmission is a result of sex is a prejudice, rather than an empirical finding. The assumption that transmission through various non-sexual routes is low is a result of not looking for evidence that would demonstrate such transmission and ignoring any evidence that comes to light, which it usually does inadvertently.[41]

But the evidence for iatrogenic, or healer-caused, infection does exist, although it is often greeted by denial. As recently as 2007, the World Health Organization maintained that the reuse of syringes without sterilization accounts for 2.5 percent of new HIV infections in Africa, but a 2003 study by David Gisselquist in the *International Journal of STD and AIDS* found that up to 40 percent of HIV infections in Africa had been caused by contam-inated needles used during medical treatment.[42] Even the con-servative WHO estimate translates to hundreds of thousands of infections.

Infections that are more common in the West than in the Global South drive mental-disease rates too, beginning with influenza. Americans think of the flu as an ailment of temperate Western climes, but influenza struck one of every five hospitalized African respiratory patients between 2006 and 2010, and one of every ten outpatients. It drives significant morbidity and mortality in Africa,[43] and in fact, Africans suffer more complications than Western patients. Elderly South Africans with influenza, for example, are four times more likely to die than their U.S. counterparts.[44] Administering vaccines to prevent influenza would greatly reduce the related risk of acquired schizophrenia, especially in newborns and the young, as detailed in chapter 2. Similarly, vaccines against the GAS infections that cause PANDAS, as established in chapter 3, could ward off anorexia, Tourette's, and OCD.

Medicines with borders

There is as yet no preventive against *T. gondii,* nor a vaccine against the hepatitis C virus, which goes hand in hand with depression; up to seven of every ten people with hepatitis C suffer from depression.[45] Nor is there a preventive for the sleeping sickness that breeds paranoia and murderous aggression.

But even if these vaccines and antibacterials existed, they would probably not benefit people of the Global South. Vaccines against influenza and antibiotics for GAS infections do exist, but they are hard to come by in the developing world. How hard? No one seems to know; a 2014 survey report of thirty-one African countries concluded that "influenza vaccines and antiviral drugs are available in many countries in Africa but coverage estimates are low and remain largely unknown."

When available, they are prohibitively expensive. When they are affordable, they are sometimes shunned by the people who desperately need them. The medically damaging injection practices and, especially, the use of ethically suspect research have fomented a loss of trust in vaccines in Nigeria. Much of the news coverage focuses on the contention by suspicious Africans that Western vaccines spread HIV and cause sterility.[46] These fears may seem unfounded to some, but they are based on a well-documented contemporary history of harms at the hand of white and Western-trained physicians.

In March 2000, Werner Bezwoda, a cancer researcher at South Africa's Witwatersrand University, was fired after conducting medical experiments involving giving very high doses of chemotherapy to black breast-cancer patients without obtaining informed consent. Dr. Michael Swango was ultimately convicted of murder after pleading guilty to killing three American patients with lethal injections of potassium, but he is also suspected in the deaths of sixty others, mostly in Zimbabwe and Zambia during the 1980s and '90s. In 1995, Richard McGown, a Scottish anesthesiologist practicing in Zimbabwe, was accused of five murders and convicted in the deaths of two infant patients whom he had injected with lethal doses of morphine. Wouter Basson, the former head of Project Coast, South Africa's chemical and biological weapons unit under apartheid, was charged with killing hundreds of black citizens of South Africa and Namibia from 1979 to 1987, many via injected poisons. He was tried but not convicted by an apartheid-holdover judge in a South African court, even though his lieutenants testified in detail and with consistency about the medical crimes they conducted against blacks. Malicious research agendas, such as the Project Coast division that vowed to create agents to selectively harm or sterilize black Africans in the guise of vaccines, are well documented. In 2015, the South African medical association censured Basson for the killings that took place under his direction during apartheid.[47]

Moreover, the widely publicized CIA perversion of vaccination programs as fronts for covert operations such as the search for Osama bin Laden and other political schemes has done much to feed Third World distrust of Westerners proffering injections. At least one CIA sham vaccination program *encouraged* the spread of infection by providing only one injection of a three-dose protocol, an inadequate treatment that made people believe they were protected against disease when they in fact were not.[48]

The practical result of all these reckless mistreatments is unambiguous: suspicious patients avoid care, and this iatrophobia, or fear of physicians, means that "conquered" diseases such as polio are seeing a resurgence on the African continent.[49] Even when vaccinations are delivered by the most dedicated health-care workers, poverty makes treatment in the developing world fraught with risk.[50] Infection control to prevent the spread of disease is difficult or impossible when there is limited access to clean water and no access to the antiseptics and cleaning agents that we take for granted in the West.

Given these varied challenges, what would be the smart move to protect the developing world from infectious diseases that may destroy minds, from the ailments spread by worms and tsetse flies to HIV and influenza?

Obviously, affordable antibiotics and psychoactive drugs must be made available. Clean water and the construction of toilets can do much to eliminate sources of infection and to damp virulence, as it denies microbes easy access to hosts. But simpler, cheaper pharmaceutical approaches could also play a role, including drugs like aspirin,[51] which protects the brain via its anti-inflammatory effects, suggests Michael Berk of Australia's Deakin University School of Medicine: "Aspirin can reduce oxidative stress and protect against oxidative damage. Early evidence suggests there are beneficial effects of aspirin in preclinical and clinical studies in mood disorders and schizophrenia." Moreover, Berk notes, "Epidemiological data suggest that high-dose aspirin...

one of the oldest agents in medicine, is a potential new therapy for a range of neuropsychiatric disorders."[52]

In neglected lands teeming with untamed infectious threats and unaddressed disease, there is much room for improvement utilizing both classic public-health measures and sophisticated infectious-disease strategies of the sort analyzed in chapter 6.

But it is a mistake to think that when Westerners address these threats to physical and mental health, we are helicoptering in just to save the bodies and minds of the downtrodden. All our medical fates are inextricably linked, and by treating disease abroad, we help to save ourselves.

Afterword

A few months after this book went to press, reports began circulating of a "new" infectious disease threat: the Zika virus. It was discovered in 1947 among rhesus monkeys in Uganda's Zika forest and had moved to humans by 1952. But before 2007, it was found only in Africa and Asia.

In May 2015, Zika surfaced in Brazil, where it infected 1.3 million people. Because it has struck regions of the world without adequate disease surveillance, we still don't know all of its medical consequences.[1] We do know that its recent spread has been rapid: within nine months it appeared in eighteen countries and territories in Latin America and the Caribbean, and travelers brought cases home to Texas, Puerto Rico, Hawaii, and Illinois.[2]

From the beginning, public health organizations have called for calm and warned against conspiracy theories, but what scientists have learned in the ensuing months is ominous.

By February 1, 2016, when the World Health Organization pronounced the burgeoning Zika virus a "public-health emergency of international concern," the measured language veiled the nearest thing to panic that the agency allows itself. Only three other disasters have earned this label: the 2009 H1N1 epidemic, the 2014 Middle Eastern polio resurgence, and the 2014 Ebola epidemic.[3]

But unlike the other three events, Zika threatens more than our physical health. Like many other infections, it can generate or encourage mental and cognitive disorders.

The World Health Organization explained that Zika virus is spread mostly by *Aedes* mosquitoes, especially *Aedes aegypti*. Sexual transmission from men to women has also been documented in the U.S. and elsewhere, and the virus persists for an unknown period in semen.[4] The usual symptoms of Zika disease include mild fever, skin rashes, muscle and joint pain, conjunctivitis, and "malaise." These last for two to seven days, but likely complications — Guillain-Barré syndrome and microcephaly in infants (small heads and underdeveloped brains) — have risen with cases of the disease.[5]

It causes only a mild rash in most adults, but fetuses can suffer stillbirth, microcephaly, and eye malformations.[6] A report in the *New England Journal of Medicine* indicted Zika as the cause of microcephaly after it analyzed the virus's entire genome. "Microscopic examination revealed that brain cells were destroyed due to infection with the virus. While it can't be definitive proof, it may present the most compelling evidence to date that congenital brain malformations associated with Zika virus infection in pregnancy are a consequence of viral replication in the fetal brain," Tatjana Avšič Županc of Slovenia's University of Ljubljana told *New Scientist*.[7] The infection causes the brain to develop abnormally, which can result in microcephaly.

Eighty-five percent of those with microcephaly suffer significant cognitive limitations.[8] But even Zika-infected children who escape microcephaly suffer limitations. These limitations can include learning disabilities that range from the minor to the significant, speech delays, seizures, movement and balance problems, short stature, and facial anomalies.[9]

Prominent scientists told the *New York Times* that Zika damage was comparable to that seen in children whose mothers were infected with rubella during pregnancy in the 1964–65 epidemic.[10] They were born with deafness, blindness, and mental problems[11] ranging from brain swelling to mental retardation. Children's brains still pay a heavy cognitive price for Zika infection because the virus directly threatens the young for the same reason that other neglected tropical diseases, or NTDs, cause mental and cognitive derangement: fully 86 percent of a newborn's metabolic budget[12] goes into building its brain, but viruses and other pathogens drain this energy by feeding on tissues and by diverting energy from their human hosts to crank out copies of themselves. Some infections can also infest the digestive tract, where they siphon off nutrients and iron. Because building a brain and fighting off pathogens are both metabolically costly tasks, brain development suffers and varying mental and cognitive deficits such as reduced attention span and lower IQ scores result.[13]

Moreover, Zika causes devastating mental disorders by attacking the brains of fetuses or exposing them to attack by the maternal immune system, "friendly fire" that can lead to a lifetime of cognitive and mental disability.[14] Decades of research illuminates how infections that attack the developing fetal brain can result in mental illness.

Such brain damage is not as rare as once thought.[15] In March 2016, the *New England Journal of Medicine* published a study by Brazilian and American researchers revealing that 29 percent of women who had ultrasound examinations after positive tests for the Zika virus carried fetuses that were later plagued by "grave outcomes." Neither is the brain damage confined to exposures during only one trimester,[16] as was widely reported.[17] Another report demonstrated a mechanism for such brain damage: in vitro experiments show that the virus "targets and destroys" those fetal cells destined to become the brain's cortex, and fetuses are affected in all three trimesters.[18] Experts fear that Zika places "even infants who appear normal at birth...at higher risk for mental illnesses later in life," according to a *New York Times* article. "The consequences of this go way beyond microcephaly."[19]

Guillain-Barré syndrome may also emerge, an assortment of alarming, even life-threatening, symptoms that come on quickly and are caused by temporary slowing of nerve conduction. The brain receives slower, fewer signals from the body, resulting in a dangerous loss of some muscle function, which can lead to the cessation of breathing. The affected person also loses sensation and receives aberrant nerve signals that result in unpleasant tingling, "crawly," and even painful sensations that can be emotionally traumatic and necessitate mental-health therapy. Recovery can take anywhere from a few weeks to a few years.[20]

So Zika is both a physical and a mental disease, but as I explained in chapter 1, we wear Cartesian blinders in allegiance to a false mental/physical divide. This often prevents us from recognizing that diseases like Zika evoke both physical and mental problems.

Fellow Travelers

Anthony Fauci, director of the National Institute of Allergy and Infectious Diseases, wrote in the *New England Journal of Medicine* that "dengue hit with a vengeance in the '90s. Then we had West

Nile in 1999, chikungunya in 2013, and lo and behold, now we have Zika in 2015 and 2016.... This is a disturbing, remarkable pattern."[21]

The ubiquitous news coverage portrays Zika as an exceptional tropical disorder, but its migration to more than twenty American states[22] is part of a recent pattern as it joins the panoply of NTDs that have recently slipped over to the West, including the Big Five: Chagas disease, cysticercosis, toxocariasis, toxoplasmosis, and trichomoniasis.[23] At least 1,500 to 2,000 neurocysticercosis cases have been diagnosed in the United States when MRIs of patients brought to emergency rooms with sudden epilepsy or fainting revealed that their brains were irregularly studded with tapeworms. At least 330,000 U.S. citizens have Chagas disease, and estimates range as high as one million. This chronic, silent parasitic infection leads to fatal heart or intestinal damage in two of every five sufferers, and it also causes intellectual slowing.[24]

Climate change is thought to be a factor in the Western spread,[25] because many microbes function only within a narrow temperature range, and parasite life cycles often require heat. But meteorological events also escalate risk. The insects that carry Chagas disease proliferated in Louisiana after Hurricane Katrina in 2005; mosquito territories are expanding with rising temperatures; and U.S. Geological Survey scientists have warned that "hazardous bacteria and fungi hitchhike across the Atlantic on [15,000-feet-high] North African dust plumes" to scatter the pathogens of the developing world over our yards and playgrounds.[26] Moreover, the *Aedes aegypti* mosquitoes,[27] which disseminate Zika, dengue fever, chikungunya, and yellow fever,[28] are spreading more widely.

The U.S. needs no global warming to lay out the welcome mat for such diseases because it already boasts temperatures that are warmer than those in most of the affluent West, such as northern Europe. "The U.S. is somewhat unusual in being a wealthy nation much of whose population lives in very warm, humid regions," Stan Cox, a senior scientist at the Land Institute, told the *Washington Post* in July 2015.[29]

Treatment Implications

So Zika is just the latest NTD newcomer to flout etiologic and geographic borders to threaten our brains and sap our intellectual abilities. What will we do about it?

Medications would normally play an important role, but as chapter 7 notes, the pharmaceutical antimicrobials pipeline is drying up, and the industry has largely abandoned the development of antibiotics, the number of which has decreased over the past twenty years.

This makes vaccine development and controlling the mosquito population critically important, especially because the same mosquitoes transmit Zika, chikungunya, and dengue viruses.[30]

A number of institutions are rising to the challenge, including the Sabin Vaccine Institute, which is testing vaccines in Brazil and Gabon. Closer to home, Peter Hotez, MD, dean of the National School of Tropical Medicine at Baylor College of Medicine in Houston, is developing vaccines with funding from the U.S. and Japanese governments and from the Gates Foundation, which has already funded some much-needed vaccines. Meanwhile, Hotez and others lobby for a greater investment in fighting NTDs like Zika at home and abroad.

From the contagion in both the developing world and U.S. citizens, to the changes in our climate, to the already sickened ethnic enclaves within our borders, treatment and prevention are not optional. Self-interest demands that we address Zika and other NTDs, because these are now U.S. diseases. Our medical interdependence makes them everyone's problem.

Acknowledgments

I remain especially grateful to those who from this work's inception kindly gave their expertise and valuable time to share with me the daunting complexities of their work. These include Paul Ewald, Susan Swedo, E. F. Torrey, Robert Yolken, Thomas Insel, and Carl Bell.

Portions of this book began life as my master's thesis at Columbia University, which meant that as I investigated the new data and avenues of research pertaining to infectious sources of mental illness, I was fortunate to have the advice of science seminar leaders in Columbia University's MA program in science journalism. Marguerite Holloway, author of *The Measure of Manhattan* and associate professor and director of Science and Environmental Journalism, gave her generous support. Both she and Jonathan Weiner, Maxwell M. Geffen Professor of Medical and Scientific Journalism at Columbia University Graduate School of Journalism and Pulitzer Prize–winning author, gave valued critical feedback to this book in its embryo state. Others at Columbia who generously shared their expertise and feedback include Robert Klitzman, director of the university's Center for Bioethics; Dean of Social Science Alondra Nelson; Professor David Sulzer; Ian Lipkin, director of the Center for Infection and Immunity; Sara Davis; and Carolina Cebrian.

Khadija Pierce, senior law and ethics associate at Harvard Law School, and Sheri Fink of the *New York Times* and author of *Five Days at Memorial* gave valuable feedback and support. So did

Joshua Prager, Heather Butts, and my friends and fellow scribes of the Invisible Institute, founded by Annie Murphy Paul and Alissa Quart, who have proved trusted advisers and beloved friends. These pillars of support include Kaja Perina, Susan Cain, Abby Ellin, Tom Zoellner, Wendy Paris, Christine Kenneally, Randi Hutter Epstein, Catherine Orenstein, Elizabeth DeVita-Raeburn, Maia Szalavitz, Stacy Sullivan, Paul Raeburn, Gretchen Rubin, Judith Matloff, Lauren Sandler, Ada Calhoun, and Gary Bass.

The original insights of Philip Alcabes, author of the brilliant *Dread: How Fear and Fantasy Have Fueled Epidemics from the Black Death to Avian Flu,* and of Alex Dajkovic, of the Institut Curie in Paris, were invaluable.

I am deeply grateful to the UNLV's Black Mountain Institute, and, in particular, to Carol C. Harter, Richard Wiley, Joseph Langdon, and Maritza White, for providing me with a home in a community of stellar writers. I thank former justice of the Nevada Supreme Court Miriam Shearing, who funded my fellowship at BMI, not only for her material support but for the gift of getting to know her as a charming, modest, but extremely effective legal pioneer.

I remain grateful for the keen judgment of my wonderful agent Lisa Bankoff and my wise, witty lawyer Zick Rubin. I am thrilled by the opportunity to thank my knowledgeable and insightful editor, Tracy Behar, who provided the close attention and organizational genius from which this work benefited. I am also very grateful to Jean Garnett and Genevieve Nierman, whose superb editing enhanced this book's organization and conformation to style, to Peggy Freudenthal, and for Tracy Roe's medical expertise and grammatical acumen.

I somehow completed this work without the support of my beloved and devoted husband, Ron DeBose, just one of the countless voids his passing has left in my life. But I've had the crucial support of Irene K. Billips, Dora Kearsley, Doris Brooks,

Crosby Kearsley Jr., Lois Friend, Donna and Tom Harman, Garth Fagan, Edgar Jackson, Libertad Matos, Shuly Adams, David and Sandie Smith, Janet Taylor, Jeff Vincent, Marcia Cassaboom, Matt and Annie Cox, Elaine Fox, Linda Schrader Jones, Eva Winkler, Kirsten Everett, Mamie Humphries, Betty Williams Collins, Jack Anderson, Cathy Wilson, Theresa Canada, Robert Taylor, Vincent Anderson, Ronnie Allen, Gail Wright Sirmans, Val McPherson, Cathleen Kehoe, Ron Buford, Bruce Jacobs, Andrew Ostergren, and my friends in the Calvary support group. They had much to do with making this book a reality.

Last but definitely not least, I am blessed in Kate, Eric, and Theresa, my sisters and brother, and I miss Pete more than words can say.

Notes

Chapter 1: Germ Theory Redux

1. John Cornwell, "Slaves to American Medicine," *Times of London Sunday Times Magazine* (with a sidebar by Harriet A. Washington), September 10, 2006.
2. This paresis patient was impaired in a manner similar to the one John Cornwell describes. I encountered him in the 1970s on the wards of the hospital where I volunteered in Rochester, New York.
3. "General Paresis," Medline.com; see also B. J. Beck, "Mental Disorders Due to a General Medical Condition," in *Massachusetts General Hospital Comprehensive Clinical Psychiatry*, ed. T. A. Stern et al. (Philadelphia: Elsevier Mosby, 2008), chapter 21.
4. Robert C. Benchley, "The Most Popular Book of the Month," in *Of All Things* (New York: Henry Holt, 1922), 187.
5. "What Was the Truth About the Madness of George III?," BBC News, April 15, 2013. See also R. E. Kendell, "The Distinction Between Mental and Physical Illness," *British Journal of Psychiatry* 178, no. 6 (June 2001).
6. M. Worboys, *Spreading Germs: Disease Theories and Medical Practice in Britain, 1865–1900* (Cambridge: Cambridge University Press, 2008).
7. E. F. Torrey and Robert Yolken, "Could Schizophrenia Be a Viral Zoonosis Transmitted from House Cats?," *Schizophrenia Bulletin* 21, no. 2 (1995).
8. Howard Robinson, "Dualism," in *The Stanford Encyclopedia of Philosophy*, ed. Edward N. Zalta (Fall 2003).
9. W. D. Hart, "Dualism," in *A Companion to the Philosophy of Mind*, ed. Samuel Guttenplan (Oxford: Blackwell, 1996), 265–67.
10. G. B. Risse, *Mending Bodies, Saving Souls: A History of Hospitals* (Oxford: Oxford University Press, 1990), 56.
11. Roy Porter, *Mind-Forg'd Manacles: A History of Madness in England from the Restoration to the Regency* (London: Athlone, 1987).
12. Michel Foucault, "Madness and Society," in *Aesthetics, Method and Epistemology*, ed. James D. Faubion (New York: New Press, 1998), 558.

13. Elliot S. Valenstein, "Debating Lunacy," *New York Times*, May 3, 2014.
14. Roy Porter, "Willis, Francis (1718–1807)," *Oxford Dictionary of National Biography* (Oxford: Oxford University Press, 2004); online edition, http://odnb2.ifactory.com/view/article/29578/29578. See also Foucault, "Madness and Society," 337–38.
15. Foucault, "Madness and Society," 337.
16. Jean L. Cooper and Angelika S. Powell, "King George's Illness— Porphyria," University of Virginia, http://people.virginia.edu/~jlc5f/charlotte/porphyria.html.
17. "About Porphyria," American Porphyria Association, http://www.porphyriafoundation.com/about-porphyria.
18. Timothy J. Peters and Allan Beveridge, "The Madness of King George III: A Psychiatric Re-Assessment," *History of Psychiatry* 21, no. 1 (March 2010): 20–37.
19. Anne Digby, "Changes in the Asylum: The Case of York, 1777–1815," *Economic History Review New Series* 36, no. 2 (May 1983): 218–39.
20. Benjamin Rush, *Medical Inquiries and Observations upon the Diseases of the Mind* (Philadelphia: Kimber and Richardson, 1812).
21. Paul E. Kopperman, "'Venerate the Lancet': Benjamin Rush's Yellow Fever Therapy in Context," *Bulletin of the History of Medicine* 78 (2004): 539–74; C. J. Tsay, "Julius Wagner-Jauregg and the Legacy of Malarial Therapy for the Treatment of General Paresis of the Insane," *Yale Journal of Biological Medicine* 86, no. 2 (2013): 245–54; Digby, "Changes in the Asylum."
22. Rush, *Medical Inquiries and Observations*; see also Harriet A. Washington, *Medical Apartheid* (New York: Doubleday, 2007), 181–82.
23. Harriet A. Washington, "The Cleansing Fire: Malaria Therapy at the Rockefeller Institute," www.metropolisofscience.org.
24. Deborah Hayden, *Pox: Genius, Madness, and the Mysteries of Syphilis* (New York: Basic Books, 2003).
25. Ibid; see also Joel Braslow, *Mental Ills and Bodily Cures: Psychiatric Treatment in the First Half of the Twentieth Century* (Berkeley: University of California Press, 1997).
26. Kendell, "The Distinction Between Mental and Physical Illness"; see also Tsay, "Julius Wagner-Jauregg."
27. Hayden, *Pox: Genius, Madness.*
28. Kendell, "The Distinction Between Mental and Physical Illness"; Tsay, "Julius Wagner-Jauregg."
29. Kat McGowan, "The Second Coming of Sigmund Freud," *Discover*, March 6, 2014, http://discovermagazine.com/2014/april/14-the-second-coming-of-sigmund-freud.
30. Lainie Friedman Ross, "Review of *Useful Bodies: Humans in the Service of Medical Science in the Twentieth Century*," *Perspectives in Biology and Medicine* 48, no. 2 (Spring 2005): 312–14.
31. Gretchen Vogel, "Malaria as a Lifesaving Therapy," *Science* 342 (November 8, 2013): 686.

32. Joel T. Braslow, "Effect of Therapeutic Innovation on Perception of Disease and the Doctor-Patient Relationship: A History of General Paralysis of the Insane and Malaria Fever Therapy, 1910–1950," *American Journal of Psychiatry* 152 (1995): 660–65.

33. John F. Mahoney, R. C. Arnold, and Ad Harris, "Penicillin Treatment of Early Syphilis—a Preliminary Report," *American Journal of Public Health* 33, no. 12 (1943): 1387–91. See also Tsay, "Julius Wagner-Jauregg."

34. Worboys, *Spreading Germs*.

35. Irvine Loudon, *The Tragedy of Childbed Fever* (New York: Oxford University Press, 2000), 6.

36. Creutzfeldt-Jakob Disease Foundation, "Possible Symptoms," http://www.cjdfoundation.org/possible-symptoms.

37. Mary Kilbourne Matossian, *Poisons of the Past: Molds, Epidemics, and History* (New Haven, CT: Yale University Press, 1991).

38. A. Woolf, "Witchcraft or Mycotoxin? The Salem Witch Trials," *Clinical Toxicology* 38, no. 4 (2000): 457–60.

39. American Psychiatric Association, *Diagnostic and Statistical Manual of Mental Disorders*, 4th ed. (Washington, DC: American Psychiatric Association, 2013).

40. Chun Siong Soon et al., "Unconscious Determinants of Free Decisions in the Human Brain," *Nature Neuroscience* 11 (2008): 543–45, doi:10.1038/nn.

41. John-Dylan Haynes and Geraint Rees, "Decoding Mental States from Brain Activity in Humans," *Nature Reviews Neuroscience* 7 (July 2006): 523–34, doi:10.1038/.

42. Stanislas Dehaene and Lionel Naccache, "Towards a Cognitive Neuroscience of Consciousness: Basic Evidence and a Workspace Framework," *Cognition* 79 (April 2001): 1–37.

43. Woo-kyoung Ahn, Caroline C. Proctor, and Elizabeth H. Flanagan, "Mental Health Clinicians' Beliefs About the Biological, Psychological, and Environmental Bases of Mental Disorders," *Cognitive Science* 33, no. 2 (2009): 147–82, doi:10.1111/j.1551-6709.2009.01008.x.

44. Tanya Marie Luhrmann, "Beyond the Brain," *Wilson Quarterly* (Summer 2012): 34.

Chapter 2: The Fetus as Battleground

1. Treatment Advocacy Center, "Dr. E. Fuller Torrey Talks About His Loved One" (video), https://www.youtube.com/watch?v=bWX13jlVL0k.

2. National Institute of Mental Health, "What Are the Symptoms of Schizophrenia?," www.nimh.nih.gov/health/publications/schizophrenia/what-are-the-symptoms-of-schizophrenia.shtml.

3. Miriam Spering et al., "Efference Copy Failure During Smooth Pursuit Eye Movements in Schizophrenia," *Journal of Neuroscience* 33, no. 29 (July 17, 2013): 11779–87.

4. L. G. Ledgerwood, P. W. Ewald, and G. M. Cochran, "Genes, Germs, and Schizophrenia: An Evolutionary Perspective," *Perspectives in Biology and Medicine* 46 (2003): 17–48; see also J. O. Davis and J. A. Phelps, "Twins

with Schizophrenia: Genes or Germs?," *Schizophrenia Bulletin* 21, no. 1 (1995): 13–18.

5. S. Bölte et al., "The Roots of Autism and ADHD Twin Study in Sweden (RATSS)," *Twin Research and Human Genetics* 17, no. 3 (February 2014): 164–76.

6. S. Maiti, "Ontogenetic De Novo Copy Number Variations (CNVS) as a Source of Genetic Individuality: Studies on Two Families with MZD Twins for Schizophrenia," *PLoS One* 6, no. 3 (March 2011).

7. Emma L. Dempster et al., "Disease-Associated Epigenetic Changes in Monozygotic Twins Discordant for Schizophrenia and Bipolar Disorder," *Human Molecular Genetics* (2011), http://hmg.oxfordjournals.org/content/early/2011/09/22/hmg.ddr416.short.

8. Davis and Phelps, "Twins with Schizophrenia."

9. Paul H. Patterson, *Infectious Behavior: Brain-Immune Connections in Autism, Schizophrenia, and Depression* (Cambridge, MA: MIT Press, 2013), 17, 36.

10. Davis and Phelps, "Twins with Schizophrenia."

11. Ibid.

12. Herbert Goldenberg and Irene Goldenberg, *Family Therapy: An Overview* (Independence, KY: Cengage Learning, 2012), 114. See also Frieda Fromm-Reichmann, *Principles of Intensive Psychotherapy* (Chicago: University of Chicago Press, 1960).

13. Tanya Marie Luhrmann, "Beyond the Brain," *Wilson Quarterly* (Summer 2012): 29–34.

14. Douglas Fox, "The Insanity Virus," *Discover*, November 8, 2010.

15. Ibid.

16. Paolo Fusar-Poli and Pierluigi Politi, "Paul Eugen Bleuler and the Birth of Schizophrenia," *American Journal of Psychiatry* 165 (2008): 1407.

17. Edwin Fuller Torrey and Judy Miller, *The Invisible Plague: The Rise of Mental Illness from 1750 to the Present* (New Brunswick, NJ: Rutgers University Press, 2007).

18. Richard Noll, "Historical Review: Autointoxication and Focal Infection Theories of Dementia Praecox," *World Journal of Biological Psychiatry* 5, no. 2 (May 2004): 66–72.

19. Richard Noll, "Kraepelin's 'Lost Biological Psychiatry'? Autointoxication, Organotherapy and Surgery for Dementia Praecox," *History of Psychiatry* 18 (September 2007): 301–20.

20. Pamela Jones, "Appendicostomy (Malone Procedure; Antegrade Colonic Enema Procedure)," http://www.crouse.org/health/PIB/Appendicostomy.

21. Jeffrey Masson, *The Assault on Truth: Freud's Suppression of the Seduction Theory* (New York: Farrar, Straus, and Giroux, 1984), 55–106; 233–50.

22. Jeffrey Masson, "Freud and the Seduction Theory: A Challenge to the Foundations of Psychoanalysis," *Atlantic*, February 1, 1984. See also Peter Gay, *Freud: A Life for Our Time* (New York: W. W. Norton, 1988), 84.

23. Arij Ouweneel, *Freudian Fadeout: The Failings of Psychoanalysis in Film Criticism* (Jefferson, NC: McFarland, 2012).

24. Lawrence K. Altman, *Who Goes First?: The Story of Self-Experimentation in Medicine* (Oakland: University of California Press, 1998).
25. Richard Noll, "Infectious Insanities, Surgical Solutions: Bayard Taylor Holmes, Dementia Praecox and Laboratory Science in Early 20th-Century America, Part 1," *History of Psychiatry* 17 (2006): 299–311. See also J. Althaus, "On Psychoses After Influenza," *Journal of Mental Science* 39 (1893): 163–76.
26. Richard Noll, "Infectious Insanities, Surgical Solutions: Bayard Taylor Holmes, Dementia Praecox and Laboratory Science in Early 20th-Century America, Part 2," *History of Psychiatry* 18 (2007): 301–20.
27. United States Census Bureau, "World Population: Historical Estimates of World Population," www.census.gov/population/international/data/worldpop/table_history.php.
28. Michael Bresalier, "'A Most Protean Disease': Aligning Medical Knowledge of Modern Influenza, 1890–1914," *Medical History* 56 (October 2012): 481–510.
29. Bertrand Dawson, "An Address on the Future of the Medical Profession: Being the Cavendish Lecture Delivered before the West London Medico-Chirurgical Society on July 4th," *British Medical Journal* 2, no. 39 (July 1918): 56–60.
30. "The Influenza Outbreak," *Journal of the American Medical Association* (*JAMA*) 71 (October 1918): 1138.
31. Karl A. Menninger, "Psychoses Associated with Influenza—1. General Data: Statistical Analysis," *JAMA* 72, no. 4 (January 1919).
32. Bresalier, "'A Most Protean Disease.'"
33. Ibid.
34. S. West, "An Address on Influenza," *Lancet* 143, no. 3687 (April 1894): 1047–52.
35. W. Harris, "The Nervous System in Influenza," *Practitioner* (August 1907): 85.
36. J. Althaus, *Influenza: Its Pathology, Symptoms, Complications, and Sequels* (London: Longmans, 1892), 13–20.
37. B. W. Richardson, "Epidemic Neuroparesis," *Asclepiad* 9 (1892): 19–37. See also B. W. Richardson, "Influenza as an Organic Nervous Paresis," *Asclepiad* 8 (1891): 178–79.
38. Bresalier, "'A Most Protean Disease,'" 499.
39. However, diagnostic tests on the appropriated corpses of affected sufferers have failed to establish a certain link between encephalitis lethargica and influenza; see "The Influenza Pandemic of 1918," at http://virus.stanford.edu/uda/.
40. R. C. Dale et al., "Encephalitis Lethargica Syndrome: 20 New Cases and Evidence of Basal Ganglia Autoimmunity," *Brain* 127, no. 1 (2004): 21–33.
41. The astonishing but temporary promise of levodopa, an ultimately futile treatment used by Oliver Sacks, is the riveting, albeit brief, exception and is discussed in his book *Awakenings* (New York: Vintage Books, 1990).

42. R. H. Yolken and E. F. Torrey, "Are Some Cases of Psychosis Caused by Microbial Agents? A Review of the Evidence," *Molecular Psychiatry* 13 (2008): 470–79.
43. Fox, "The Insanity Virus."
44. Michael Winerip, "Schizophrenia's Most Zealous Foe," *New York Times*, February 22, 1998.
45. Treatment Advocacy Center, "Homelessness: One of the Consequences of Failing to Treat Individuals with Severe Mental Illnesses," Backgrounder Briefing Paper, March 2011, http://www.treatmentadvocacycenter.org/resources/consequences-of-lack-of-treatment/homelessness/1379.
46. Thomas Szasz, *Ceremonial Chemistry* (Garden City, NY: Anchor, 1974).
47. Fox, "The Insanity Virus."
48. Ibid.
49. Ibid.
50. Ibid.
51. Ibid.
52. Ibid.
53. Ibid.
54. Ibid.
55. Ian Lipkin, interview with the author, April 1, 2013.
56. E. Fuller Torrey and Robert H. Yolken, "Could Schizophrenia Be a Viral Zoonosis Transmitted from House Cats?," *Schizophrenia Bulletin* 21, no. 2 (1995).
57. E. Fuller Torrey and Robert H. Yolken, "*Toxoplasma gondii* and Schizophrenia," *Emerging Infectious Diseases* (November 2003), http://wwwnc.cdc.gov/eid/article/9/11/03-0143.htm.
58. E. Fuller Torrey, John J. Bartko, and Robert H. Yolken, "*Toxoplasma gondii* and Other Risk Factors for Schizophrenia: An Update," *Schizophrenia Bulletin* 38, no. 3 (May 2012).
59. Yolken and Torrey, "Are Some Cases of Psychosis Caused by Microbial Agents?"
60. Ibid., 471.
61. R. H. Yolken, F. B. Dickerson, and E. Fuller Torrey, "Toxoplasma and Schizophrenia," *Parasite Immunology* 31 (November 2009): 711.
62. A. S. Brown et al., "Maternal Exposure to Toxoplasmosis and Risk of Schizophrenia in Adult Offspring," *American Journal of Psychiatry* 162, no. 4 (2005): 767–73. See also P. B. Mortensen et al., "*Toxoplasma Gondii* as a Risk Factor For Early-Onset Schizophrenia: Analysis of Filter Paper Blood Samples Obtained at Birth," *Biological Psychiatry* 61 (2007): 688–93.
63. Yolken, Dickerson, and Torrey, "Toxoplasma and Schizophrenia," 706–15.
64. Ibid., 708.
65. Ibid., 707.
66. Ibid., 708.
67. Ibid., 711–12.
68. Ibid., 712.

69. "Brain Morphology and Schizophrenia: Enlarged Ventricles," University of Toronto neurowiki website, http://neurowiki2013.wikidot.com/individual:brain-morphology.

70. C. Gaser et al., "Ventricular Enlargement in Schizophrenia Related to Volume Reduction of the Thalamus, Striatum, and Superior Temporal Cortex," *American Journal of Psychiatry* 161, no. 1 (January 2004): 154–56.

71. Fox, "The Insanity Virus."

72. The famine known as the Dutch Hunger Winter was intentionally caused when a German blockade cut off food shipments affecting 4.5 million people and killing as many as 22,000. This was undertaken in retaliation for instances of Dutch resistance to Nazism. Anthony Sas, "Holland's 'Hunger Winter' of 1944–45," *Military Review* 63, no. 9 (September 1983): 24–32. See also *Uitzending Gemist, Vroeger & Zo De hongerwinter—1944* (video), http://www.npo.nl/vroeger-zo/01-06-2012/NPS_1197941.

73. Laura C. Schulz, "The Dutch Hunger Winter and the Developmental Origins of Health and Disease," *Proceedings of the National Academy of Sciences* 107, no. 39 (2010): 16757–58.

74. Adi Narayan, "Side Effects of 1918 Flu Seen Decades Later," *Time*, October 12, 2009.

75. Thomas F. McNeil, E. Cantor-Graae, and D. R. Weinberger, "Relationship of Obstetric Complications and Differences in Size of Brain Structures in Monozygotic Twin Pairs Discordant for Schizophrenia," *American Journal of Psychiatry* 157, no. 2 (February 2000): 203–12.

76. Pak C. Sham et al., "Schizophrenia Following Pre-Natal Exposure to Influenza Epidemics Between 1939 and 1960," *British Journal of Psychiatry* 160 (1992).

77. A. Brown et al., "Serologic Evidence of Prenatal Influenza in the Etiology of Schizophrenia," *Archives of General Psychiatry* 61 (August 2004): 774–80.

78. Sham, "Schizophrenia Following Pre-Natal Exposure to Influenza." See also J. McGrath and D. Castle, "Does Influenza Cause Schizophrenia? A Five-Year Review," *Australian and New Zealand Journal of Psychiatry* 29, no. 1 (March 1995): 23–31.

79. Thomas H. Maugh II, "Paul Patterson Dies at 70; Caltech Neuroscientist," *Los Angeles Times*, July 18, 2014.

80. High-throughput sequence animation from Sadava et al., *Life: The Science of Biology*, 9th edition, Sinauer Associates, http://www.sumanasinc.com/webcontent/animations/content/highthroughput2.html. Accessed December 17, 2012.

Chapter 3: Growing Pains

1. Susan Swedo, interview with the author, March 15, 2013.

2. The names of Jane and Seth have been changed, as have some details of their story, in order to protect their privacy.

3. According to the Centers for Disease Control and Prevention (CDC), only 1 to 3 percent of people with streptococcal throat infections develop

ARF; thus, the incidence of ARF in the United States is thought to be
about 0.5 per 100,000 patients between five and seventeen years of age.

4. Varnada Karriem-Norwood, "Understanding Rheumatic Fever: The
Basics," WebMD, March 14, 2014, http://www.webmd.com/a-to-z-guides/
understanding-rheumatic-fever-basics.
5. Ibid.
6. The antigens found include B lymphocyte antigen D8/17.
7. A. K. Khanna, "Presence of a Non-HLA B Cell Antigen in Rheumatic
Fever Patients and Their Families as Defined by a Monoclonal Antibody,"
Journal of Clinical Investigation 83, no. 1710 (1989).
8. E. Hollander et al., "B Lymphocyte Antigen D8/17 and Repetitive
Behaviors in Autism," *American Journal of Psychiatry* 156 (1999): 317–20;
Susan Swedo et al., *Journal of the American Academy of Child and Adolescent
Psychiatry* 34, no. 307 (1995); *American Journal of Psychiatry* 154, no. 110
(1997); *American Journal of Psychiatry* 154, no. 402 (1997).
9. Susan Swedo, interview with the author, March 15, 2013.
10. Tourette Syndrome fact sheet, Office of Communications and Public
Liaison, National Institute of Neurological Disorders and Stroke, http://
www.ninds.nih.gov/disorders/tourette/detail_tourette.htm.
11. Some details of her experience, including Bertha's real name, have been
changed in order to protect the family's privacy.
12. "Eating Disorders Statistics," National Association of Anorexia Nervosa
and Associated Disorders, http://www.anad.org/get-information/
about-eating-disorders/eating-disorders-statistics/.
13. J. L. Jarry and F. J. Vaccariono, "Eating Disorder and Obsessive-Compulsive
Disorder: Neurochemical and Phenomenological Commonalities,"
Journal of Psychiatry and Neuroscience 21, no. 1 (January 1996): 36–48.
14. Mae S. Sokol, "Infection-Triggered Anorexia Nervosa," *Eating Disorders
Review* 12, no. 5 (September/October 2001).
15. National Institute of Mental Health, "Eating Disorders: About More Than
Food," http://www.nimh.nih.gov/health/publications/eating-disorders
-new-trifold/eating-disorders-pdf_148810.pdf.
16. S. J. Crow et al., "Increased Mortality in Bulimia Nervosa and Other
Eating Disorders," *American Journal of Psychiatry* 166 (2009): 1342–46.
17. Patrick F. Sullivan, "Course and Outcome of Anorexia Nervosa and
Bulimia Nervosa," *American Journal of Psychiatry* 152, no. 7 (July 1995):
1073–74.
18. Ibid.
19. NIMH, "Eating Disorders: About More Than Food."
20. M. S. Sokol, "Infection-Triggered Anorexia Nervosa in Children: Clinical
Description of Four Cases," *Journal of Child and Adolescent Psychopharmacology*
10, no. 2 (2000): 133–45.
21. Susan E. Swedo et al., "High Prevalence of Obsessive-Compulsive
Symptoms in Patients with Sydenham's Chorea," *American Journal of
Psychiatry* 146, no. 2 (1989): 246–49.

22. Susan E. Swedo, James F. Leckman, and Noel R. Rose, "From Research Subgroup to Clinical Syndrome: Modifying the PANDAS Criteria to Describe PANS (Pediatric Acute-Onset Neuropsychiatric Syndrome)," *Pediatrics and Therapeutics* (2012).

23. William C. Robertson Jr., "Chorea in Children," Medscape, http://emedicine.medscape.com/article/1181993-overview. Accessed April 2, 2013.

24. "How Cavity-Causing Microbes Invade the Heart," *ScienceDaily*, June 28, 2011.

25. M. E. Pichichero, "The PANDAS Syndrome," *Advances in Experimental Medicine and Biology* 634 (2009): 205–16.

26. Harriet Washington, "The Infection Connection," *Psychology Today*, July 1, 1999.

27. Harriet Washington, "A New Kind of Mental Disease, a New Kind of Person," presentation delivered at Columbia University Department of Anthropology, July 3, 2013. See also Ian Hacking, *Historical Ontology* (Cambridge, MA: Harvard University Press, 2004), 168, 169.

28. Mary MacIntosh, "The Homosexual Role," *Social Problems* (1968).

29. Hacking, *Historical Ontology*, 164.

30. Ibid.

31. Thomas Ungar and Stephanie Knaack, "The Hidden Medical Logic of Mental Health Stigma," *Australian and New Zealand Journal of Psychiatry* 47, no. 7 (July 2013): 611–12.

32. Patrick W. Corrigan and Amy C. Watson, "Stop the Stigma: Call Mental Illness a Brain Disease," *Schizophrenia Bulletin* 30, no. 3 (2004): 477–79.

33. Ungar and Knaack, "The Hidden Medical Logic," 611.

34. Paul Ewald, *Plague Time: The New Germ Theory of Disease* (New York: Anchor, 2002), xvi; see also D. H. Thom et al., "Association of Prior Infection with Chlamydia Pneumonia and Angio-Graphically Demonstrated Coronary Heart Disease," *JAMA* 268 (1992): 68–72; and C. R. Meier et al., "Antibiotics and Risk of Subsequent First-Time Myocardial Infarction," *JAMA* 281 (1999): 427–31.

35. Ewald, *Plague Time*, xvi.

36. Although Swedo has proposed a nomenclature change from PANDAS to PANS (pediatric acute-onset neuropsychiatric syndrome) in order to include other disease triggers, PANDAS remains the established and most prevalent usage.

37. How do we even know that PANDAS is an autoimmune disorder? In 1957, Ernst Witebsky, a German immunologist who had helped to characterize the A and B blood groups before fleeing Nazi Germany for the University of Buffalo, established the criteria for labeling a disease autoimmune. First, you must identify the antibody of the known target (autoantigen), then evoke the disease in animals by transferring the antibodies from one animal to another, a disease route called passive transfer; see E. Witebsky et al., *JAMA* 164 (1957): 1439–47; and N. R. Rose and C. Bona,

"Defining Criteria for Autoimmune Diseases (Witebsky's Postulates Revisited)," *Immunology Today* 14 (September 1993): 426–30.

38. In 2012, Swedo recast PANDAS as PANS, which implicates any infectious agent, not just GAS, as a possible causative agent and which focuses heavily on anxiety and behavioral problems as criteria for diagnosis. I have referred to PANDAS throughout the book because it is so similar and it is the most familiar rendition of the syndrome.

39. The *Diagnostic and Statistical Manual of Mental Disorders IV,* published in 2000, was actually a quasi–fifth edition, as it incorporated major revisions; see "*DSM-5* Publication Date Moved to May 2013," press release from the American Psychiatric Association, December 10, 2009.

40. The *DSM-5* Neurodevelopmental Disorders Work Group, quoted in Eve Herold, "Commentary Takes Issue with Criticism of New Autism Definition: *DSM- 5* Experts Call Study Flawed," press release, American Psychiatric Association, March 27, 2012.

41. Kristine M. Kulage, Arlene M. Smaldone, and Elizabeth G. Cohn, "How Will *DSM-5* Affect Autism Diagnosis? A Systematic Literature Review and Meta-Analysis," *Journal of Autism and Developmental Disorders* (2014).

42. Jonathan Metzl, *The Protest Psychosis: How Schizophrenia Became a Black Disease* (Boston: Beacon, 2011). See also J. C. West et al., "Race/Ethnicity Among Psychiatric Patients: Variations in Diagnostic and Clinical Characteristics," *Journal of Lifelong Learning in Psychiatry* 4 (2006): 48–56; and interview with Carl C. Bell, director, Institute for Juvenile Research and Professor, Department of Psychiatry and School of Public Health, University of Illinois at Chicago, http://sites.nationalacademies.org/DBASSE/CLAJ/DBASSE_081977#.UXMqqILBCj4.

43. Robert V. Guthrie, *Even the Rat Was White: A Historical View of Psychology* (Boston: Allyn and Bacon, 2003). See also Stephen Jay Gould, *The Mismeasure of Man* (New York: W. W. Norton, 1993).

44. Marilynn Elias, "Conflicts of Interest Bedevil Psychiatric Drug Research," *USA Today,* June 3, 2009. See also Harriet A. Washington, *Deadly Monopolies* (New York: Doubleday, 2011).

45. Ferris Jabr, "Beyond Symptoms," *Scientific American* (May 2013): 17.

46. "*DSM-5* Development," American Psychiatric Association (2011), http://www.dsm5.orghttp://www.dsm5.org/pages/default.aspx.

47. Nicholas Bakalar, "More Diseases Pinned on Old Culprit: Germs," *New York Times,* May 17, 2005.

48. Ian Lipkin, interview with the author, April 1, 2013.

49. James E. Bowman and Robert F. Murray Jr., *Genetic Variation and Disorders in Peoples of African Origin* (Baltimore: Johns Hopkins University Press, 1998); author's personal communications with Dr. Bowman.

50. V. Jacomo, P. Kelly, and D. Raoult, "Natural History of Bartonella Infections (an Exception to Koch's Postulate)," *Clinical and Diagnostic Laboratory Immunology* 9, no. 1 (2002): 8–18.

51. Judith Hooper, "A New Germ Theory," *Atlantic,* February 1, 1999.

52. D. Nash et al., "The Outbreak of West Nile Virus Infection in the New York City Area in 1999," *New England Journal of Medicine* 344, no. 24 (June 2001): 1807–14.

53. K. Ambroz, "Improving Quantitation Accuracy for Western Blots," *Image Analysis* (September 2006).

54. W. Ian Lipkin, "Biographical Sketch," Center for Infection and Immunity, http://cii.columbia.edu/team.aspx?l8psqK&cid=WYUHOo.

55. Ian Lipkin, interview with the author, April 1, 2013.

56. Joanna Kempner, Clifford S. Perlis, and Jon F. Merz, "Forbidden Knowledge," *Science* 307, no. 5711 (February 2005): 854.

57. J. W. Konturek, "Discovery by Jaworski of *Helicobacter pylori* and Its Pathogenetic Role in Peptic Ulcer, Gastritis and Gastric Cancer," *Journal of Physiology and Pharmacology* 54 (2003): 23–41.

58. For an entrancing history of self-experimentation among physicians, I again refer you to Lawrence K. Altman, *Who Goes First?: The Story of Self-Experimentation in Medicine* (Oakland: University of California Press, 1998).

59. B. J. Marshall, "History of the Discovery of *C. pylori*," in *Campylobacter pylori in Gastritis and Peptic Ulcer Disease*, ed. M. J. Blaser (New York: Igaku-Shoin, 1989), 7.

60. Kimball Atwood, "*H. pylori*, Plausibility, and Greek Tragedy: The Quirky Case of Dr. John Lykoudis," *Science-Based Medicine* (blog), March 26, 2010.

61. Ibid.

62. Reza Malekzadeh et al., "Treatment of *Helicobacter pylori* Infection in Iran: Low Efficacy of Recommended Western Regimens," *Archives of Iranian Medicine* 7, no. 1 (2004): 1–8.

63. Mark Kidd and Irvin M. Modlin, "A Century of *Helicobacter pylori*," *Digestion* 59, no. 1 (1998): 1–15.

64. Centers for Disease Control, "Knowledge about Causes of Peptic Ulcer Disease, United States, March–April 1997," *Morbidity and Mortality Weekly Report* 46, no. 42 (1997): 985–87.

65. M. Sweet, "Smug as a Bug," *Sydney Morning Herald*, August 2, 1997.

66. *H. pylori* also underwent a bit of an identity crisis. It was originally, and ungrammatically, dubbed *Campylobacter pylorides* and subsequently emended to *Campylobacter pylori*, which is better Latin but still biologically incorrect because the bacterium does not fit within the genus *Campylobacter*. It belongs to its own genus, *Helicobacter*.

67. NIH Consensus Conference, "*Helicobacter pylori* in Peptic Ulcer Disease, NIH Consensus Development Panel on *Helicobacter pylori* in Peptic Ulcer Disease," *JAMA* 272 (1994): 65–69.

68. L. M. Brown, "*Helicobacter pylori*: Epidemiology and Routes of Transmission," *Epidemiology Review* 22, no. 2 (2000): 283–97.

69. Michelle Stacey, "The Fall and Rise of Kilmer McCully," *New York Times*, August 10, 1997. See also Gary Taubes, "The Game of the Name," *Discover*, January 23, 2003.

70. Christopher Snowdon, *Velvet Glove, Iron Fist: A History of Anti-Smoking* (New York: Little Dice, 2009).
71. Tucker Cummings, "The History of Cervical Cancer," http://www.ehow.com/about_5554342_history-cervical-cancer.html.
72. "Williams took Sims to task for pronouncements he continued to make about the sexual health and, by implication, the morality of black women. For example, Sims had reported that '60 percent' of Negro women had uterine cancer (a disease then associated with early and frequent sexual contact) or uterine fibroids." Harriet A. Washington, *Medical Apartheid*, first digital draft edition, 68. Also see Helen Buckler, *Dr. Dan* (Boston: Little, Brown, 1954), 183, 191; cited in Eugene P. Link, "The Civil Rights Activities of Three Great Negro Physicians," *Journal of Negro History* 52, no. 3 (1967): 169–84.

Chapter 4: Gut Feelings

1. George C. Williams, *Adaptation and Natural Selection* (Princeton, NJ: Princeton University Press, 1996).
2. Gina Kolata, "In Good Health? Thank Your 100 Trillion Bacteria," *New York Times*, June 13, 2012.
3. Gregory G. Dimijian, "Pathogens and Parasites: Insights from Evolutionary Biology," *Baylor University Medical Center Proceedings* 12 (1999): 175–87.
4. F. Guarner and J. Malagelada, "Gut Flora in Health and Disease," *Lancet* 361 (2003): 512–19.
5. Adam Hadhazy, "Think Twice: How the Gut's 'Second Brain' Influences Mood and Well-Being," *Scientific American*, April 30, 2014.
6. Rob Stein, "Gut Bacteria Might Guide the Workings of Our Minds," *Shots: Health News*, NPR, November 18, 2013.
7. Martin J. Blaser, "Who Are We? Indigenous Microbes and the Ecology of Human Diseases," *EMBO Reports* 7 (2006): 956–60, http://embor.embopress.org/content/7/10/956.
8. "Mitochondrial DNA," National Library of Medicine Genetics Home Reference, http://ghr.nlm.nih.gov/mitochondrial-dna.
9. Paul R. Burkholder and Ilda Mcveigh, "Synthesis of Vitamins by Intestinal Bacteria," *Proceedings of the National Academy of Sciences of the USA*, 28 (7), 285–89.
10. University of Rochester Medical Center, "Amid the Murk of 'Gut Flora,' Vitamin D Receptor Emerges as a Key Player," *Science Daily*, July 8, 2010. Also see Blaser, "Who Are We?"
11. Martin J. Blaser, *Missing Microbes: How the Overuse of Antibiotics Is Fueling Our Modern Plagues* (New York: Henry Holt, 2014).
12. Vlaams Instituut voor Biotechnologie, "Mission and Objectives," http://www.vib.be/en/about vib/organization/Pages/Mission-and-goals.aspx.
13. The organization that conducted the gene census is Metagenomics of the Human Intestinal Tract; see Junjie Qin et al., "A Human Gut Microbial Gene Catalogue Established by Metagenomic Sequencing," *Nature* 464 (March 2010): 59–65.
14. Denise Grady, "Study Sees Bigger Role for Placenta in Newborns' Health," *New York Times*, May 21, 2014.

15. Kjersti Aagaard et al., "The Placenta Harbors a Unique Microbiome," *Science Translational Medicine* 6 (May 2014): 237.

16. "Life Map: Embryonic Development and Stem Cell Compendium; Neural Crest Development and Stem Cells," http://Discovery.Lifemapsc. Com/In-Vivo-Development/Neural-Crest.

17. J. R. Seckl and M. J. Meaney, "Glucocorticoid Programming," *Annals of the New York Academy of Sciences* 1032 (2004): 63–84.

18. Jeroen Raes, "The Gut Flora: You and Your 100 Trillion Friends: Jeroen Raes at TEDx Brussels," https://www.youtube.com/watch?v=Af5qUxl1ktI. See also figure 2 in Dimijian, "Pathogens and Parasites."

19. Hadhazy, "Think Twice."

20. Blaser, *Missing Microbes.*

21. Joseph's name and some details of his story have been changed to protect his and his family's privacy.

22. "History of Autism," WebMD, http://www.webmd.com/brain/autism/history-of-autism.

23. "ASD Data and Statistics," CDC.gov, http://www.cdc.gov/ncbddd/autism/data.html.

24. Hanne Jakobsen, "A Farewell to Asperger's Syndrome," *ScienceNordic,* May 19, 2012.

25. Ian Hacking, "Making Up People," *London Review of Books* 38 (August 2006): 16–26.

26. Ian Hacking, "The Looping Effects of Human Kinds," in *Causal Cognition: A Multi-Disciplinary Debate,* eds. Dan Sperber, David Premack, and Ann James Premack (New York: Oxford University Press, 1995), 351–83.

27. Philip Alcabes, *Dread: How Fear and Fantasy Have Fueled Epidemics from the Black Death to Avian Flu* (New York: Public Affairs, 2010), Kindle edition.

28. Jessica Stoller-Conrad, "Probiotic Therapy Alleviates Autism-like Behaviors in Mice," Caltech, December 5, 2013.

29. Elaine Y. Hsiao et al., "Microbiota Modulate Behavioral and Physiological Abnormalities Associated with Neurodevelopmental Disorders," *Cell* 155, no. 7 (December 19, 2013): 1451–63.

30. Hadhazy, "Think Twice."

31. John Ayto, ed., *Oxford Dictionary of English Idioms,* 3rd ed. (Oxford: Oxford University Press, 2010), 1863.

32. Alison C. Bested, Alan C. Logan, and Eva M. Selhub, "Intestinal Microbiota, Probiotics and Mental Health: From Metchnikoff to Modern Advances: Part II—Contemporary Contextual Research," *Gut Pathogens* 5, no. 3 (2013).

33. Ibid.

34. M. Lyte, J. J. Varcoe, and M. T. Bailey, "Anxiogenic Effect of Subclinical Bacterial Infection in Mice in the Absence of Overt Immune Activation," *Physiological Behavior* 65 (1998): 63–68; see also Bested, "Intestinal Microbiota."

35. M. Maes et al., "In Depression, Bacterial Translocation May Drive Inflammatory Responses, Oxidative and Nitrosative Stress (O&NS), and

Autoimmune Responses Directed Against O&NS-Damaged Neoepitopes," *Acta Psychiatrica Scandinavica* 127, no. 5 (May 2013): 344–54.

36. Linda Geddes, "Gut Bacteria May Contribute to Autism," *New Scientist*, June 7, 2010.

37. Sally Ozonoff et al., "A Prospective Study of the Emergence of Early Behavioral Signs of Autism," *Journal of the American Academy of Child and Adolescent Psychiatry* 49, no. 2 (March 2010): 256–66.

38. Also, in 2011, Bruce Beutler shared the Nobel Prize in Physiology or Medicine for his work demonstrating how the bacterial LPS generate toxins. Beutler, director of the Center for the Genetics of Host Defense at the University of Texas, showed how cytokines goad the powerful responses by the immune-system LPS. See Yong-Chen Lu, Wen-Chen Yeh, and Pamela S. Ohas, "LPS/TLR4 Signal Transduction Pathway," *Cytokine* 42, no. 2 (May 2008): 145–51.

39. S. M. Finegold et al., "Gastrointestinal Microflora Studies in Late-Onset Autism," *Clinical Infectious Disease* 35 (2002): S6–S16.

40. R. H. Sandler et al., "Short-Term Benefit from Oral Vancomycin Treatment of Regressive-Onset Autism," *Journal of Child Neurology* 15 (2000): 429–35.

41. Tori Rodriguez, "Gut Bacteria May Exacerbate Depression," *Scientific American*, October 17, 2013.

42. T. W. Stone, "Neuropharmacology of Quinolinic and Kynurenic Acids," *Pharmacology Review* 45 (1993): 309–79.

43. D. Benton, C. Williams, and A. Brown, "Impact of Consuming a Milk Drink Containing a Probiotic on Mood and Cognition," *European Journal of Clinical Nutrition* 61 (2007): 355–61. Also see A. V. Rao et al., "A Randomized, Double-Blind, Placebo-Controlled Pilot Study of a Probiotic in Emotional Symptoms of Chronic Fatigue Syndrome," *Gut Pathology* 1, no. 6 (2009), and M. Messaoudi et al., "Assessment of Psychotropic-Like Properties of a Probiotic Formulation (*Lactobacillus helveticus* R0052 and *Bifidobacterium longum* R0175) in Rats and Human Subjects," *British Journal of Nutrition* 105 (2011): 755–64.

44. F. Bäckhed, "Host Responses to the Human Microbiome," *Nutritional Reviews* 70, no. 1, Supplement S14-7 (August 2012).

45. National Institutes of Health, "Human Microbiome Project: Program Snapshot," http://commonfund.nih.gov/hmp/index, July 14, 2014.

46. Kate Murphy, "In Some Cases, Even Bad Bacteria May Be Good," *New York Times*, October 31, 2011.

47. National Institutes of Health, "Human Microbiome Project."

48. T. Ding and P. D. Schloss, "Dynamics and Associations of Microbial Community Types Across the Human Body," *Nature* (April 16, 2014).

49. Alejandro Reyes et al., "Viruses in the Faecal Microbiota of Monozygotic Twins and Their Mothers," *Nature* 466 (July 2010): 334–38.

50. Kolata, "In Good Health?"

51. John Gever, "Obesity Rejected as Psychiatric Diagnosis in *Diagnostic and Statistical Manual of Mental Disorders*, 5th Edition," *MedPage Today*, May 29, 2010, http://www.medpagetoday.com/MeetingCoverage/APA/20381.

52. Evelyn Attia et al., "Feeding and Eating Disorders in the *Diagnostic and Statistical Manual of Mental Disorders,* 5th Edition," *American Journal of Psychiatry* 170 (November 2013): 1237–39.

53. Julia Lurie, "Measles Cases in the US Are at a 20-Year High. Thanks, Anti-Vaxxers," *Mother Jones,* May 29, 2014.

54. "The Centenary of Panum," *American Journal of Public Health* 36 (July 1946).

55. For this quotation, as well as for much of the discussion about measles, I am indebted to Hugh Pennington's column "Why Can't Doctors Be More Scientific?," *London Review of Books* 26, no. 13 (July 2004): 28–29.

56. "Measles Encephalitis," in *Jawetz, Melnick, and Adelberg's Medical Microbiology,* ed. George Brooks et al. (New York: Lange, 2010), 586.

57. Pennington, "Why Can't Doctors Be More Scientific?"

58. W. J. Bellini et al., "Subacute Sclerosing Panencephalitis: More Cases of This Fatal Disease Are Prevented by Measles Immunization Than Was Previously Recognized," *Journal of Infectious Diseases* 192, no. 10 (2005): 1686–93.

59. Michael Pollan, "Some of My Best Friends Are Germs," *New York Times,* May 15, 2013.

60. I. Youngster et al., "Oral, Capsulized, Frozen Fecal Microbiota Transplantation for Relapsing *Clostridium difficile* Infection," *JAMA* 312, no. 17 (November 2014): 1772–78 (erratum in *JAMA* 313, no. 7 [February 2015]: 729). See also Mandy Oaklander, "Fecal Transplants May Soon Be Available in a Pill," *Time,* October 11, 2014.

Chapter 5: Microbial Culture

1. Alexandra Smith, "Long Beach Journal; Eyes That Saw Horrors Now See Only Shadows," *New York Times,* September 8, 1989, http://www.nytimes.com/1989/09/08/us/long-beach-journal-eyes-that-saw-horrors-now-see-only-shadows.html. Also in 1980, the American Psychiatric Association officially changed the diagnosis of "hysterical neurosis, conversion type" to conversion disorder, but *hysteria* retains its colloquial currency.

2. M. Sierra and G. E. Berrios, "Towards a Neuropsychiatry of Conversive Hysteria," *Cognitive Neuropsychiatry* 4 (1999): 267–87.

3. Ibid.

4. Susan Dominus, "What Happened to the Girls in Le Roy," *New York Times Magazine,* March 7, 2012.

5. Wen-Shing Tseng, "From Peculiar Psychiatric Disorders Through Culture-Bound Syndromes to Culture-Related Specific Syndromes," *Transcultural Psychiatry* 43, no. 4 (December 2006): 554–76; Andrew N. Wilner, "An Explanation for Mass Hysteria?," *Medscape Neurology,* July 11, 2012.

6. Johan J. Mattelaer and Wolfgang Jilek, "Koro—the Psychological Disappearance of the Penis," *Journal of Sexual Medicine* 4, no. 5 (2007): 1509–15.

7. Vivian Afi Dzokoto and Glenn Adams, "Understanding Genital-Shrinking Epidemics in West Africa: Koro, Juju, or Mass Psychogenic Illness?," *Culture, Medicine, and Psychiatry* 29, no. 1 (March 2005): 53–78.

8. A. Kleinman and Tsung-Yi Lin, *Normal and Abnormal Behavior in Chinese Culture* (Dordrecht, Holland: Reidel, 1980), 237–72.

9. Wen-Shing Tseng, "From Peculiar Psychiatric Disorders."

10. Dzokoto and Adams, "Understanding Genital-Shrinking Epidemics."

11. Janis H. Jenkins, "Ethnopsychiatric Interpretations of Schizophrenic Illness: The Problem of Nervios within Mexican-American Families," *Culture, Medicine, and Psychiatry* 12 (1988): 301–29.

12. Ibid., 319.

13. Ibid.

14. John B. Schorling and J. Terry Saunders, "Is 'Sugar' the Same as Diabetes? A Community-Based Study Among Rural African-Americans," *Diabetes Care* 2, no. 3 (2000): 330–34.

15. R. Bell, *Holy Anorexia* (Chicago: University of Chicago Press, 1985). Also see Caroline Giles Banks, "'Culture' in Culture-Bound Syndromes: The Case of Anorexia Nervosa," *Social Science and Medicine* 34, no. 8 (1992): 867–84.

16. Banks, "'Culture' in Culture-Bound Syndromes."

17. Ibid., 869.

18. Pierluigi Gambetti, "Kuru," *Merck Manual Home Edition*, http://www.merckmanuals.com/home/brain_spinal_cord_and_nerve_disorders/prion_diseases/kuru.html.

19. For a description of kuru, see Robert Klitzman, *The Trembling Mountain: A Personal Account of Kuru, Cannibals, and Mad Cow Disease* (New York: Plenum, 1998), 51–52.

20. Lawrence K. Altman, "The Doctor's World: The Mystery of Balanchine's Death Is Solved," *New York Times*, May 8, 1984.

21. Alvin F. Poussaint, "Is Extreme Racism a Mental Illness?," *Western Journal of Medicine* 176, no. 1 (January 2002): 4.

22. Ibid.

23. Harriet A. Washington, "Mortal Lessons: HSPH Faculty Confront a Uniquely American Scourge," *Harvard Public Health Review* (September 1998).

24. "Major predictors of sporting gun ownership include having parents who owned guns and currently having friends and neighbors with guns. Individuals surrounded by gun owners tend to want guns themselves"; see David Hemenway, "Risks and Benefits of a Gun in the Home," *American Journal of Lifestyle Medicine* 5, no. 6 (2011): 502–11. Also see David Hemenway, *Private Guns, Public Health* (Ann Arbor: University of Michigan Press, 2006).

25. Fox Butterfield, "Crime Fighting's About-Face," *New York Times*, January 19, 1997.

26. Elizabeth Norton, "Is Prison Contagious?," *Science/AAAS News*, June 26, 2014.

27. Gary Slutkin, "Violence Is a Contagious Disease," in *The Contagion of Violence* (Washington, DC: National Academies Press, 2011).
28. Brandon Keim, "Is It Time to Treat Violence Like a Contagious Disease?," *Wired,* January 18, 2013.
29. Mark Schaller, "Parasites, Behavioral Defenses, and the Social Psychological Mechanisms Through Which Cultures Are Evoked," *Psychological Inquiry* 17 (2006): 96–101.
30. Ilan Shrira, "Guns, Germs, and Stealing: Exploring the Link Between Infectious Disease and Crime," *Evolutionary Psychology* 11, no. 1 (2011): 270–87.
31. Jacqueline Weaver, "Researchers Discover Animals Will Shun Others with Infectious Diseases," *Yale Bulletin and Calendar* 28, no. 7 (October 1999).
32. The Advocacy Project, *Srebrenica Genocide* (blog), "Bosnia Death Toll: 104,732 (Minimum)," March 30, 2011, http://srebrenicagenocide.blogspot.com/2011/03/bosnia-death-toll-104732.html.
33. Rick Chillot, "Do I Make You Uncomfortable?," *Psychology Today,* November 5, 2013.
34. R. Thornhill and C. L. Fincher, "The Parasite-Stress Theory of Sociality and the Behavioral Immune System," in *Evolutionary Perspectives in Social Psychology,* ed. L. Welling, V. Zeigler-Hill, and T. K. Shackelford (New York: Springer, 2014).
35. Shrira, "Guns, Germs, and Stealing."
36. Kipling D. Williams and Lisa Zadro, "Ostracism: The Early Detection System," draft of Presentation at the 7th Annual Sydney Symposium of Social Psychology, *The Social Outcast: Ostracism, Social Exclusion, Rejection, and Bullying.*
37. Poussaint, "Is Extreme Racism a Mental Illness?" Also see Gordon W. Allport, *The Nature of Prejudice: 25th Anniversary Edition* (New York: Basic Books, 1979).
38. Philip Alcabes, *Dread: How Fear and Fantasy Have Fueled Epidemics from the Black Death to Avian Flu* (New York: Public Affairs, 2010), Kindle edition.
39. Harriet A. Washington, *Medical Apartheid* (New York: Doubleday, 2007), 194.
40. Clarence Lusane, *Hitler's Black Victims: The Historical Experiences of European Blacks, Africans and African Americans During the Nazi Era* (New York: Routledge Crosscurrents in African American History, 2002), 140.
41. Stormfront, "Race—the Brutal Truth!," http://expeltheparasite.com/books/race-the-brutal-truth/.
42. Carlos David Navarrete and Daniel M. T. Fessler, "Disease Avoidance and Ethnocentrism: The Effects of Disease Vulnerability and Disgust Sensitivity on Intergroup Attitudes," *Evolution and Human Behavior* 27 (2006): 270–82.
43. Fergal Keane, *Season of Blood: A Rwandan Journey* (New York: Penguin Books, 1997), 9.

44. Ibrahim M. Omer, "Are Genetic Differences at the Root of the Tutsi-Hutu Rwandan Conflict?," Genetic Literacy Project, http://www.genetic literacyproject.org/2013/08/05/are-genetic-differences-at-the-root -of-the-tutsi-hutu-rwandan-conflict/.

45. Chillot, "Do I Make You Uncomfortable?"

46. "World's Funniest Taste Test," https://www.youtube.com/watch?v=Yh -BLE8v9Wk.

47. "Toxo: A Conversation with Robert Sapolsky about Toxoplasmosis," Edge Foundation video, June 19, 2011, http://www.sott.net/article/230158 -Toxo-A-Conversation-with-Robert-Sapolsky-about-Toxoplasmosis.

48. Kathleen McAuliffe, "How Your Cat Is Making You Crazy," *Atlantic*, February 6, 2012.

49. James Harbeck, "17 Disgusting Descriptions for Delicious Wines," *Week*, January 22, 2014.

Chapter 6: Winning at Evolutionary Chess

1. Jonas Ahl et al., "Bacterial Aetiology in Ventilator-Associated Pneumonia at a Swedish University Hospital," *Scandinavian Journal of Infectious Diseases* 42 (2010): 6–7.

2. H. Wunsch et al., "The Epidemiology of Mechanical Ventilation Use in the United States," *Critical Care Medicine* 38, no. 10 (2011): 1947–53.

3. At least over the short term. Because a ventilator can threaten your life too. If the air leaks from the lung into the chest wall, it can cause a pneumothorax (a collapsed lung). The elevated partial pressures of oxygen can lead to oxygen toxicity, which may injure the lungs and the brain. Blood clots and vocal-cord damage are also risks. Of course, people on ventilators are closely monitored, and these problems have medical solutions.

4. Thomas Häusler, *Viruses vs. Superbugs: A Solution to the Antibiotics Crisis?* (London: Palgrave Macmillan, 2006).

5. This was not exactly a random insight, because two of the four doctors in the study were shareholders in the company that distributed Lp299. Although Lund University's ethical board approved the study, this could be construed as a serious conflict of interest, and the investigators could hardly be considered disinterested.

6. Carl Zimmer, "Fast-Reproducing Microbes Provide a Window on Natural Selection," *New York Times,* June 26, 2007.

7. Andrew Grant, "The Big Idea That Might Beat Cancer and Cut Health-Care Costs by 80 Percent," *Discover,* September 30, 2009.

8. Deborah Gouge, "Big Pharma Abandons Antibiotics: An Opening for Small Biotech," *Seeking Alpha* (blog), May 13, 2012, http://seekingalpha .com/article/584871-big-pharma-abandons-antibiotics-an-opening -for-small-biotech.

9. John Rhodes, *The End of Plagues: The Global Battle Against Infectious Disease* (New York: St. Martin's, 2013).

10. Ross Upshur, "Ethics and Infectious Disease Bulletin of the World Health Organization," http://www.who.int/bulletin/volumes/86/8/08 -056242/en/.

11. Ibid.

12. Häusler, *Viruses vs. Superbugs.*

13. Gouge, "Big Pharma Abandons Antibiotics."

14. Adam Hadhazy, "What Comes After Antibiotics? Alternatives to Stop Superbugs," *Popular Mechanics,* December 21, 2013.

15. Zsuzsanna Jakab, *The Bacterial Challenge: Time to React, Joint Technical Report, 2008,* European Centre for Disease Prevention and Control (ECDC) and the European Medicines Agency (EMEA), http://www.ecdc.europa.eu/ en/publications/Publications/0909_TER_The_Bacterial_Challenge _Time_to_React.pdf.

16. Gouge, "Big Pharma Abandons Antibiotics."

17. Sarah J. Fentress and L. David Sibley, "The Secreted Kinase ROP18 Defends Toxoplasma's Border," *Bioessays* 33 (2011): 693–700.

18. Grant, "The Big Idea."

19. Harriet A Washington, *Living Healthy with Hepatitis C: Natural and Conventional Approaches to Recover Your Quality of Life* (New York: Dell, 2000).

20. Meera Senthilingam, "Malaria Bug May Give Mosquitoes a Super Sense of Smell," *New Scientist,* May 15, 2013.

21. Richard Dawkins, *The Extended Phenotype: The Long Reach of the Gene* (Oxford: Oxford University Press, 1982).

22. Ibid., 43.

23. Tara C. Smith, "Psychological Disorders Associated with Cerebral Malaria," *Aetiology* (blog), April 20, 2010, http://scienceblogs.com/aetiology/ 2010/04/20/psychological-disorders-associ/.

24. David Pedersen, "UI/VAMC Study Says Patient's History of Malaria May Be a Clue to Many Vietnam Vets' Psychological and Other Health Problems," Newswise, January 8, 1998, http://www.newswise.com/articles/ uivamc-study-says-patients-history-of-malaria-may-be-a-clue-to-many -vietnam-vets-psychological-and-other-health-problems.

25. Gregory G. Dimijian, "Pathogens and Parasites: Insights from Evolutionary Biology," *Baylor University Medical Center Proceedings* 12 (1999): 75–187.

26. Dawkins, *The Extended Phenotype,* 3.

27. "Up to 80 percent of people who test positive for herpes antibodies may have symptoms so mild that they fail to recognize them, or may have no symptoms at all"; Ruth Padawer, NorthJersey.com, June 26, 2005.

28. Bill Drake, "Infection Control in Hospitals," *American Society of Heating, Refrigerating and Air-Conditioning Engineers Journal* 48 (June 2006): 12.

29. J. P. Burke, "Infection Control—a Problem for Patient Safety," *New England Journal of Medicine* 348, no. 7 (2003): 651–56.

30. Drake, "Infection Control in Hospitals," 12–17.

31. Frank Strick, "The Role of Infections in Mental Illness," Environmental Illness Resource, http://www.eiresource.org.

32. Laura Landro, "Why Hospitals Want Patients to Ask Doctors, 'Have You Washed Your Hands?'" *Wall Street Journal*, September 30, 2013; Ana Pujols McKee, "Health Care's Dirty Secret: Physician's [*sic*] Don't Wash Their Hands as Often as Other Caregivers," *JC Physician* (blog), Joint Commission, September 4, 2013, http://www.jointcommission.org/jc_physician_blog/health_cares_dirty_secret/.

33. Agnes Ullmann, "Pasteur-Koch: Distinctive Ways of Thinking About Infectious Diseases," *Microbe* 2, no. 8 (2007): 383–87.

34. Landro, "Why Hospitals Want Patients to Ask Doctors."

35. Ibid.

36. Eleanor Nelsen, "Antibacterial Soap Is Fouling Up Sewage Treatment Systems," NOVA Next, June 20, 2014.

37. Drake, "Infection Control in Hospitals."

38. Jay C. Fournier et al., "Antidepressant Drug Effects and Depression Severity: A Patient-Level Meta-Analysis," *JAMA* 303, no. 1 (2010): 47–53.

39. John Kelley, "Antidepressants: Do They 'Work' or Don't They?," *Scientific American*, March 2, 2010.

40. Lennard J. Davis, "Five Reasons Not to Take SSRIs," *Obsessively Yours* (blog), January 7, 2010, https://www.psychologytoday.com/blog/obsessively-yours/201001/five-reasons-not-take-ssris.

41. In 2011 Marcia Angell, a Harvard professor and former editor of the *New England Journal of Medicine*, summarized the case against antidepressants in a dual *New York Review of Books* analysis entitled "The Epidemic of Mental Illness: Why?" and "The Illusions of Psychiatry." Within the last decade, at least four other peer-reviewed medical analyses have drawn the same conclusion, and psychologist Irving Kirsch is among the experts who have published books on the topic; his is entitled *The Emperor's New Drugs: Exploding the Antidepressant Myth*.

42. Bridget M. Kuehn, "Questionable Antipsychotic Prescribing Remains Common, Despite Serious Risks," *JAMA* 303, no. 16 (2010): 1582–84.

43. Ibid.

44. Kelley, "Antidepressants."

45. Kuehn, "Questionable Antipsychotic Prescribing."

46. Ramin Mojtabai and Mark Olfson, "National Trends in Psychotropic Medication Polypharmacy in Office-Based Psychiatry," *Archives of General Psychiatry* 67, no. 1 (2010): 26–36.

47. Harriet A. Washington, "Flacking for Big Pharma," *American Scholar* (Summer 2011).

48. Harriet A. Washington, *Deadly Monopolies* (New York: Doubleday, 2011).

49. Ross J. Tynan et al., "A Comparative Examination of the Anti-Inflammatory Effects of SSRI and SNRI Antidepressants on LPS-Stimulated Microglia," *Brain, Behavior, and Immunity* 26 (2012): 469–79.

50. Ibid.

51. Ibid.

52. V. P. Sergiev, "Directed Modulation of Host's Behavior Favouring Transmission of Pathogen," *Zhurnal mikrobiologii, epidemiologii, i immuno-*

biologii 3 (May–June 2010): 108–14. From the abstract, translated from the Russian: "It turned out that parasites use the same neuromediators for change of behavior of both mammals and hosts belonging to other animal classes. In fishes as well as in mammals, monoamines-neurotransmitters assist in brain functioning. Norepinephrine, dopamine and serotonin affect the alimentation, motion activity, aggression and social behaviour."

53. Tynan, "A Comparative Examination."
54. Melinda Wenner, "Infected with Insanity," *Scientific American* (April–May 2008): 46.
55. Washington, *Living Healthy*.
56. R. Foster, D. Olajide, and I. P. Everall, "Antiretroviral Therapy-Induced Psychosis: Case Report and Brief Review of the Literature," *HIV Medicine* 4, no. 2 (April 2003): 139–44.
57. Wenner, "Infected with Insanity," 46–47; see also Paul H. Patterson, "Pregnancy, Immunity, Schizophrenia, and Autism," *Engineering and Science* 69, no. 3 (2006): 10–21, and Paul H. Patterson, "Maternal Effects on Schizophrenia Risk," *Science* 318 (2007): 576–77.
58. Matthew S. Kayser and Josep Dalmau, "The Emerging Link Between Autoimmune Disorders and Neuropsychiatric Disease," *Journal Neuropsychiatry Clinical Neuroscience* 23, no. 1 (Fall 2011): 90–97.
59. M. S. Kayser, C. G. Kohler, and J. Dalmau, "Psychiatric Manifestations of Paraneoplastic Disorders," *American Journal of Psychiatry* 167 (2010): 1039–50.
60. Jane E. Brody, "Babies Know: A Little Dirt Is Good for You," *New York Times,* January 26, 2009.
61. D. E. Elliott et al., "Exposure to Helminthic Parasites Protect Mice from Intestinal Inflammation," *Gastroenterology* 116: A706 (1999); also see A. Agrawal, Q. M. Eastman, and D. G. Schatz, "Transposition Mediated by RAG1 and RAG2 and Its Implications for the Evolution of the Immune System," *Nature* 394 (1998): 744–51.
62. Rachel Nuwer, "Worm Therapy: Why Parasites May Be Good for You," BBC Future, April 22, 2013.
63. T. Paparrigopoulos et al., "The Neuropsychiatry of Multiple Sclerosis: Focus on Disorders of Mood, Affect and Behavior," *International Review of Psychiatry* 22, no. 1 (2010): 14–21.
64. This patient's story is described in the medical journal noted here, but I have invented the vignette's dialogue and changed some features to ensure her privacy; see A. Aggarwal et al., "Acute Psychosis as the Initial Presentation of MS," *International MS Journal* 17, no. 2 (2011): 54–57.
65. Ibid.
66. Kayser and Dalmau, "The Emerging Link."
67. Judith Hooper, "A New Germ Theory," *Atlantic,* February 1, 1999.
68. Alan S. Brown et al., "Serologic Evidence of Prenatal Influenza in the Etiology of Schizophrenia," *Archives of General Psychiatry* 61, no. 8 (2004): 774–80.
69. Hadhazy, "What Comes After Antibiotics?"

70. Ibid.
71. Laura Manuelidis, interview with the author, April 14, 2013. Also, the World Health Organization reports that "sleeping sickness was the first or second greatest cause of mortality in [Central African] communities, ahead of even HIV/AIDS," sowing dementia and killing tens of thousands, while related diseases threaten the mental health and lives of the poor throughout the Americas. See also Washington, *Deadly Monopolies*, 103.

Chapter 7: Tropical Madness

1. The names and some details have been changed and the dialogue invented, but the particulars of Acanit's story are related in R. Foster, D. Olajide, and I. P. Everall, "Antiretroviral Therapy-Induced Psychosis: Case Report and Brief Review of the Literature," *HIV Medicine* 4, no. 2 (April 2003): 139–44.
2. Sarah Steffen, "More Efforts Needed to Fight Neglected Tropical Diseases," *Deutsche Welle*, September 28, 2012. Please also see the discussions of copycat drugs in Marcia Angell, *The Truth About Drug Companies* (New York: Random House, 2009), and Harriet A. Washington, *Deadly Monopolies* (New York: Doubleday, 2011).
3. See Angell, *The Truth About Drug Companies*, and Washington, *Deadly Monopolies*, especially chapter 8, "Biocolonialism."
4. H. Wittchen and O. Riedel, "Depression and Anxiety in Parkinson's Disease: Under-Diagnosed and Undertreated," *European Neuropsychopharmacology* 21 (September 2011): S220–S221. Also see Daniel Cressy, "Psychopharmacology in Crisis as Research Funds for New Psychiatric Drugs Diminish," *Nature* (June 14, 2011).
5. CBC News, "New Psychiatric Drugs Low Priority for Pharmaceutical Firms," October 15, 2012.
6. Chiponda Chimbelu, "Pharma Patent Cliff May Lead to Research Drop-Off," *Deutsche Welle*, October 23, 2012.
7. Tatum Anderson, "Africa Rises to HIV Drug Challenge," BBC News, June 8, 2006. Also see Steffen, "More Efforts Needed."
8. Steffen, "More Efforts Needed"; see also Washington, *Deadly Monopolies*.
9. Washington, *Deadly Monopolies*, chapter 8; Deborah Gouge, "Big Pharma Abandons Antibiotics: An Opening for Small Biotech," *Seeking Alpha* (blog), May 13, 2012.
10. Gouge, "Big Pharma Abandons Antibiotics."
11. Ibid.
12. African trypanosomiasis is confined mainly to tropical Africa between 15 degrees north and 20 degrees south latitude; World Health Organization, "African Trypanosomiasis (Sleeping Sickness)," fact sheet no. 259, October 2010, http://www.who.int/mediacentre/factsheets/fs259/en/.
13. Ibid.
14. Ibid.

15. Leila Chimelli and Francesco Scaravilli, "Trypanosomiasis," *Brain Pathology* 7 (2008): 559–611.

16. Médecins sans Frontières (MSF), "Saving Lives in the Name of Vanity," January 28, 2002, http://www.msf.org/article/saving-lives-name-vanity.

17. Anne Moore, "Infectious Diseases Related to Travel; Trypanosomiasis (African Sleeping Sickness)," Centers for Disease Control Yellow Book (Atlanta: Centers for Disease Control and Prevention, 2014).

18. National Institute of Mental Health, "Sleeping Sickness," Medline Plus, http://www.nlm.nih.gov/medlineplus/ency/article/001362.htm.

19. Ibid. Also see World Health Organization, "Human African Trypanosomiasis."

20. Ann G. Sjoerdsma, *Starting with Serotonin: How a High-Rolling Father of Drug Discovery Repeatedly Beat the Odds* (Alexandria, VA: Improbable Books, 2008); MSF press release, Geneva, May 3, 2001, "Supply of Sleeping Sickness Drugs Confirmed," http://www.msf.org/article/supply-sleeping -sickness-drugs-confirmed.

21. Washington, *Deadly Monopolies*, 142–47.

22. MSF press release, "Supply of Sleeping Sickness Drugs"; also see Médecins Sans Frontières, "Saving Lives."

23. Michael Kremer, "Pharmaceuticals and the Developing World," *Journal of Economic Perspectives* 16, no. 4 (Autumn 2002): 67–90.

24. Richard Idro et al., "Cerebral Malaria: Mechanisms of Brain Injury and Strategies for Improved Neuro-Cognitive Outcomes," *Pediatric Research* 68 (2010): 267–74. See also Sumadhya D. Fernando, Chaturaka Rodrigo, and Senaka Rajapakse, "The Hidden Burden of Malaria: Cognitive Impairment Following Infection," *Malaria Journal* 9, no. 366 (2010).

25. Lawrence K. Altman, "The Doctor's World: The Mystery of Balanchine's Death Is Solved," *New York Times*, May 8, 1984.

26. Ibid.

27. "Infection, Inflammation, and Mental Illness," *Harvard Mental Health Letter*, October 1, 2009.

28. World Health Organization, "Taeniasis/Cysticercosis," fact sheet no. 376, updated May 2014, http://www.who.int/mediacentre/factsheets/fs376/en/.

29. Ibid.

30. Frank Strick, "The Role of Infections in Mental Illness," Environmental Illness Resource, http://www.eiresource.org.

31. Naresh Nebhinanil and Surendra Kumar Mattoo, "Psychotic Disorders with HIV Infection: A Review," *German Journal of Psychiatry* 16, no. 1 (2013): 43–48.

32. U.S. Department of Health and Human Services, "HIV/AIDS 101: Global Statistics," AIDS.gov, https://aids.gov/hiv-aids-basics/hiv-aids -101/global-statistics; also see World Health Organization, "AIDS Fact Sheet," http://www.who.int/mediacentre/factsheets/fs360/en.

33. Andrew C. Blalock, Sanjay Sharma, and J. Stephen McDaniel, "Anxiety Disorders and HIV Disease," in *HIV and Psychiatry: Training and Resource*

Manual, 2nd edition, ed. Kenneth Citron, Marie-Jose Brouillette, and Alexandra Beckett (Cambridge: Cambridge University Press, 2005).

34. Nebhinanil and Mattoo, "Psychotic Disorders with HIV Infection."

35. Richard A. Price, "HIV INSite Knowledge Base Chapter," HIV INSite, University of California at Los Angeles, June 1998, http://hivinsite.ucsf.edu/InSite?page=kb-04-01-03.

36. Nebhinanil and Mattoo, "Psychotic Disorders with HIV Infection." Also, Rif S. El-Mallakh, "HIV-Related Psychosis," *Journal of Clinical Psychiatry* 53, no. 8 (August 1992): 293–94.

37. Nebhinanil and Mattoo, "Psychotic Disorders with HIV Infection."

38. Ibid. Also, El-Mallakh, "HIV-Related Psychosis."

39. Nebhinanil and Mattoo, "Psychotic Disorders with HIV Infection."

40. Ibid.

41. Simon Collery, "Denial Reigns Supreme in the HIV Industry," *Don't Get Stuck with HIV* (blog), http://dontgetstuck.org/2014/07/10/denial-reigns-supreme-in-the-hiv-industry; also see "Millennium Development Goals for All, but at All Costs?," HIV in Kenya blog, July 23, 2014. Also see Andy Coghlan, "Needles, Not Sex, Drove African AIDS Pandemic," *New Scientist,* February 20, 2003.

42. David Gisselquist et al., "HIV Infections in Sub-Saharan Africa Not Explained by Sexual or Vertical Transmission," *International Journal of STD and AIDS* 13 (2002): 657–66; Harriet A. Washington, "Why Africa Fears Western Medicine," *New York Times,* July 31, 2007.

43. Mark A. Katz et al., "Influenza in Africa: Uncovering the Epidemiology of a Long-Overlooked Disease," *Journal of Infectious Diseases* 206 (2012): S1–S4. "Among 15 countries of the African Network for Influenza Surveillance and Epidemiology (ANISE), 10 percent and 22 percent of inpatient and outpatient respiratory cases, respectively, tested positive for influenza between 2006–2010"; Jazmin Duque, Meredith L. McMorrow, and Adam L. Cohen, "Influenza Vaccines and Influenza Antiviral Drugs in Africa: Are They Available and Do Guidelines for Their Use Exist?," *Public Health* 14, no. 41 (2014).

44. Duque, McMorrow, and Cohen, "Influenza Vaccines and Influenza Antiviral Drugs."

45. Sajjad Ali Memon et al., "Frequency of Depression in Chronic Hepatitis C Naïve Patients," *Pakistan Journal of Medical Sciences* 27 (July/September 2011): 780–83.

46. Peter Robison, "The CIA Stops Fake Vaccinations as Real Polio Rebounds," *Bloomberg Businessweek,* May 21, 2014.

47. Harriet A. Washington, *Medical Apartheid* (New York: Doubleday, 2007), 392; also see "Dr. Wouter Basson Found Guilty of Unprofessional Conduct," *Bulletin of the Health Professions Council of South Africa,* http://www.hpcsa-blogs.co.za/dr-wouter-basson-found-guilty-of-unprofessional-conduct/; D. L. Chandler, "South African Doctor Found Guilty of Creating Drugs, Chemicals to Kill Africans," *News One,* December 20,

2013; and also see Ina Skosana, "Truth Has Prevailed, Says Basson Victim's Wife," *Mail and Guardian,* December 18, 2013.
48. Mark Mazzetti, "U.S. Cites End to C.I.A. Ruses Using Vaccines," *New York Times,* May 20, 2014, http://www.nytimes.com/2014/05/20/us/us-cites-end-to-cia-ruses-using-vaccines.html?_r=0; also see "How the CIA's Fake Vaccination Campaign Endangers Us All," *Scientific American* 38, no. 5 (April 16, 2013).
49. John Murphy, "Polio: A Scourge of the Mid-20th Century Eludes Global Eradication and Begins to Spread as Fearful Nigerians Shun Vaccination," *Baltimore Sun,* January 4, 2004. Also see World Health Organization, "Update on Polio in Central Africa—Polio Confirmed in Equatorial Guinea, Linked to Outbreak in Cameroon," April 17, 2014, http://www.who.int/csr/don/2014_4_17polio/en/; and see S. Rushton and M. Kett, "Polio, Conflict and Distrust: A Global Public Health Emergency," *Medicine, Conflict and Survival* 30, no. 3 (2014): 143–45.
50. "Mental Health Care in the Developing World," *Psychiatric Times* (January 1, 2002), http://www.psychiatrictimes.com/articles/mental-health-care-developing-world#sthash.YOnCewEL.dpuf. Also see Washington, "Why Africa Fears Western Medicine."
51. Michael Berk et al., "Aspirin: A Review of Its Neurobiological Properties and Therapeutic Potential for Mental Illness," *BMC Medicine* 11, no. 74 (2013).
52. Ibid.

Afterword

1. Donald G. McNeil Jr., "Zika May Increase Risk of Mental Illness, Researchers Say," *New York Times,* February 18, 2016.
2. Meghan Rosen, "Rapid Spread of Zika Virus in the Americas Raises Alarm: Mosquito-Borne Disease Linked to Birth Defect Is Pushing Northward from Brazil," *Science News,* January 22, 2016, https://www.sciencenews.org/article/rapid-spread-zika-virus-americas-raises-alarm?mode=pick&context=169.
3. McNeil, "Zika May Increase Risk of Mental Illness."
4. Liz Szabo, "WHO: Sexual Transmission of Zika More Common than Thought," *USA Today,* March 8, 2016.
5. WHO Media Centre, "Zika Virus Fact Sheet," updated February 2016, http://www.who.int/mediacentre/factsheets/zika/en.
6. McNeil, "Zika May Increase Risk of Mental Illness."
7. Andy Coghlan, "Whole Zika Genome Recovered from Brain of Baby," *New Scientist,* February 10, 2016, https://www.newscientist.com/article/2077091-whole-zika-genome-recovered-from-brain-of-baby-with-microcephaly.
8. "Diseases and Conditions: Microencephaly," Mayo Clinic, http://www.mayoclinic.org/diseases-conditions/microcephaly/basics/definition/CON-20034823.

9. "Microcephaly Symptoms & Causes," Conditions + Causes, Boston's Children's Hospital http://www.childrenshospital.org/conditions-and-treatments/conditions/microcephaly/symptoms-and-causes.

10. Ibid.

11. "About Rubella," Centers for Disease Control and Prevention, http://www.cdc.gov/rubella/about/index.html.

12. M. A. Holliday, "Body Composition and Energy Needs During Growth," in F. Falkner, J. M. Tanner, eds., *Human Growth: A Comprehensive Treatise*. New York: Plenum, 1986; vol. 2: pp. 101–17.

13. Harriet A. Washington, "The Well Curve: Tropical Diseases Are Undermining Intellectual Development in Countries with Poor Health Care—And They're Coming Here Next," *American Scholar*, Autumn 2015.

14. McNeil, "Zika May Increase Risk of Mental Illness."

15. "Originally, doctors in Brazil believed that infections in the first trimester were the most dangerous, because mothers who gave birth to babies with microcephaly were usually infected then." Donald G. McNeil Jr., Catherine Saint Louis, and Nicholas St. Fleur, "Short Answers to Hard Questions About Zika Virus," *New York Times*, updated March 18, 2016.

16. W. Kleber de Oliveira, J. Cortez-Escalante, W. T. De Oliveira, et al., "Increase in Reported Prevalence of Microcephaly in Infants Born to Women Living in Areas with Confirmed Zika Virus Transmission During the First Trimester of Pregnancy—Brazil, 2015," Morb Mortal Wkly Rep 2016; 65:242–47.

17. "Originally, doctors in Brazil believed that infections in the first trimester were the most dangerous, because mothers who gave birth to babies with microcephaly were usually infected then." Donald G. McNeil Jr., Catherine Saint Louis, and Nicholas St. Fleur, "Short Answers to Hard Questions About Zika Virus," *New York Times*, updated March 18, 2016.

18. Donald G. McNeil Jr. and Catherine Saint Louis, "Two Studies Strengthen Links Between the Zika Virus and Serious Birth Defects," *New York Times*, March 4, 2016.

19. McNeil, "Zika May Increase Risk of Mental Illness."

20. Guillain-Barré Syndrome Fact Sheet, National Institute of Neurological Disorders and Stroke, http://www.ninds.nih.gov/disorders/gbs/detail_gbs.htm.

21. A. S. Fauci and D. M. Morens, "Zika Virus in the Americas—Yet Another Arbovirus Threat," *New England Journal of Medicine*, published online January 13, 2016, doi:10.1056/NEJMp1600297.

22. "To Breed, or Not to Breed: A Fearsome Outbreak Has Triggered a Debate About Birth Control," *The Economist*, January 30, 2016 [Bogotá and São Paulo].

23. Washington, "The Well Curve."

24. Brazil's average IQ is 87 (Richard Lynn and Tatu Vanhanen, *IQ and the Wealth of Nations* [Westport, CT: Praeger, 2002]), a ranking it shares with nine other countries, all in the developing world.
25. Justin Gillis, "In Zika Epidemic, a Warning on Climate Change," *New York Times,* February 20, 2016.
26. Washington, "The Well Curve."
27. Clare Wilson, "7 Ways the War on Zika Mosquitoes Could Be Won," *New Scientist,* February 2, 2016. "And in the 1960s several South American countries—including Brazil—eliminated it by spraying with DDT and urging households to get rid of breeding sites. Unfortunately the mosquitoes survived in a few locations, and after the development of a yellow fever vaccine, campaigns dwindled."
28. Ibid.
29. Rick Noack, "Europe to America: Your Love of Air Conditioning Is Stupid," *Washington Post,* July 26, 2015.
30. Rosen, "Rapid Spread of Zika Virus in the Americas Raises Alarm."

Index

adenosine monophosphate–activated
  protein kinase, 154
adenosine triphosphate (ATP), 130–31
African sleeping sickness, 231, 232–36,
  247
AIDS dementia complex, 243–44
  See also HIV/AIDS
Alcabes, Philip, 140–41
Allport, Gordon, 180
Althaus, Julius, 56
Altman, Lawrence, 168, 240
altruism, 127
Alzheimer's disease, 147–48, 222, 239
amok, 163, 164
amygdala, 162
animal models, 64–65, 68, 71, 113,
  136–38
Anopheles mosquito, 4, 200, 201–2
anorexia nervosa, 5
  culture and, 166–67
  Group A streptococci and, 6, 16–17, 33,
    86, 96
  PANDAS and, 86–87, 91–94, 98, 167
anosognosia, 40, 60
anthrax, 32
antianxiety agents, 137
antibacterial chemicals, 211
antibiotics, 196, 207
  autism and, 145, 146–47
  in developing world, 231, 237, 247, 249
  early exposure to, 133–34
  heart attack and, 103
  misuse of, 197, 221
  phage therapy vs., 223–24
  resistance to, 126, 157, 193, 194,
    196–97, 211, 223
  for schizophrenia, 75

for toxoplasmosis, 70
for ulcers, 117, 118–19, 121
antibodies, 74
  PANDAS and, 89, 90–91, 101, 160–61
  schizophrenia and, 47, 52, 73, 216
antidepressants, 93, 135, 137, 211–13
antigen, 86
antiseptic techniques, 209–10, 246
anxiety, measurement of, 136–37
apartheid, South African, 248
ASD (autism spectrum disorder), 105,
  139
Asperger's syndrome, 105
aspirin, 249–50
association, strength and consistency of,
  112
asthma, 218, 221
asylums, 17–18, 24, 27, 28
ataque de nervios, 163–64, 165–66
ATP (adenosine triphosphate), 130–31
attention deficit disorder, 70
autism, 6, 74, 138–43
  controversy over, 139–41
  DSM-5 classification of, 105, 139
  genetics and, 45, 141–42
  gut microbes and, 17, 33, 124, 129,
    137–38, 141
  influenza and, 73
  leaky gut in, 141, 143–44
  regressive-onset theory of, 145–47
  streptococcal infection and, 86, 96
  symptoms of, 138, 144–45
  vaccines and, 140, 144
autism spectrum disorder (ASD), 105,
  139
autoimmune diseases, 215–21
  gut microbes and, 33, 143, 144

autoimmune diseases *(Cont.)*
  immune response in, 64–65, 88
  See also PANDAS
autointoxication genera, 143
Aventis, 235

Bacillus anthracis, 32
bacteria, 3, 16–17
  antibiotic resistance in, 126, 157, 193, 194, 196–97, 211, 223
  beneficial, 131, 211, 223
  in biofilm, 193–94
  heart disease and, 6, 16, 96–97, 123
  intestinal, 128, 150–51
  mitochondria and, 130–31
  reproduction by, 196, 206
  See also gut microbes; pathogens; *specific species*
bacteriophages, 197, 223–24
Bacteroides fragilis, 137–38, 141
Bacteroidetes, 150
Baker, Robert A., 60
Balanchine, George, 168, 239–40
Banks, Caroline Giles, 166–67
Barker, D. J., 71
basal ganglia, 97
Bassaganya-Riera, Josep, 148
Basson, Wouter, 248
Baydoun, May, 147
Bayer, 236
Bayle, Antoine-Laurent, 27
Bayliss, William M., 134
behavior
  and infectious diseases, 36–37, 204–5
  and microbes, 8, 136–38, 142–43, 158, 174–80, 185–91, 201–3
behavioral despair test, 136–37
behavioral immune system, 174–75, 176, 179
Belshaw, Robert, 62
Benchley, Robert, 11
benzodiazepines, endogenous, 137
Berk, Michael, 249
Beveridge, Allan, 23
Bezwoda, Werner, 248
bias, 8, 30
  in *DSM-5,* 105, 106
  in prisons, 172
  See also prejudice
bifidobacteria, 148, 149

binge-eating disorder, 152
bin Laden, Osama, 249
biofilm, 193–94
biological gradient, 112
bipolar disorder, 23, 54
  genetics and, 44, 45
  influenza and, 70, 72, 73
  retroviruses and, 63–64
  seasonality of, 57–58
  toxoplasmosis and, 13, 69
birth-month effect, 57
Biss, Eula, 144
Bizzozero, Giulio, 118
Black Death, 205
Blaser, Martin J., 6, 137
Bleuler, Eugen, 52, 139
bornavirus, 5, 16, 73–74, 208
Bosnian War, 169, 178
Boyd, Mark, 30
Bradford Hill criteria, 112–13
brain
  enteric nervous system and, 4, 134–35, 137
  infectious damage of, 10–11, 74, 156, 214, 238
  "mind" and, 12
  neural disruption in, 160–61
  neuroimaging of, 61, 74
  schizophrenic, 51, 65, 70, 72, 73
Brandt, Allan M., 31
Braslow, Joel T., 31
Brockovich, Erin, 161
Bronowski, Jacob, 119
Brown, Alan S., 72–73, 213
Brown, H. Rap, 170
Brueghel, Pieter, the Younger, 85

Cahalan, Susannah, 215, 217
Camus, Albert, 158
cancer, 96
  Helicobacter pylori and, 118, 147
  human papillomavirus and, 5, 16, 75, 96, 122–23
cannibalism, 168–69, 238–39
CANS (childhood acute-onset neuropsychiatric syndrome), 103, 104
Carlat, Daniel, 213
carriers, disease, 13, 108, 176, 201, 205
Cartesian dualism, 17–19

cats and *Toxoplasma gondii*, 13–14, 204
  schizophrenia and, 52, 66–71
  tastes shaped by, 185–91
causation
  correlation vs., 91, 102–3, 106
  proof of, 106–9, 111–14, 117–23
Centers for Disease Control and
    Prevention, 121, 214
central nervous system, 133, 134
  See also brain
cerebral palsy, 84
cervical cancer, 5, 16, 75, 122–23
Chagas disease, 232–33, 255
Charcot, Jean-Martin, 159
Charlotte, Princess, 22
Charlotte, Queen of England, 20, 21
childbed fever, 32, 209
childhood acute-onset neuropsychiatric
    syndrome (CANS), 103, 104
chlamydia, 205
Chlamydophila pneumoniae, 6, 16, 97, 123
chlorine, 206
cholera, 108, 205
civet cats, 186–87
civet musk, 190
Claviceps purpurea, 4, 85
clergy vs. doctors, 17–18, 24–27, 28
Clostridium bacteria, 96–97, 146, 157
coffee, gourmet, 185–87, 188
collectivism, 183–84
Collery, Simon, 246
Columbia University, 109
Columbus, Christopher, 27
commensalism, 128, 131
concordance, twin, 43–44, 45, 47
contagion vs. infection, 172–73
conversion disorder, 159, 160–62
Cornwell, John, 9, 11
correlation vs. causation, 91, 102–3, 106, 107
Cotton, Henry, 54
Cox, Stan, 256
Crepaz-Keay, David, 40–41
Creutzfeldt-Jakob disease
  cause of, 33, 108, 123, 222, 239–40
  cultural practices and, 168–69
crime, violent, 41, 178–79
Crohn's disease, 217, 218
crypsis, 145
culture, 171
  and bias, 105, 106

collectivistic vs. individualistic, 183–84
  mental disorders related to, 162–69
  microbial shaping of, 8, 158, 174–80
  schizophrenia outcome and, 42
cytochrome P-450 enzymes, 245
cytokines, 55, 64, 70, 143
cytomegalovirus, 47, 50, 51–52, 64, 73–74

danse macabre, 83, 98
Darré, Richard Walther, 182
Dawkins, Richard, 127, 202
definitive proof, 111, 113, 114
deinstitutionalization, 58–59
Dekkers, Marijn, 236
de Kruif, Paul, 125–26
delusional disorder, 170
dementia
  Alzheimer's, 147–48, 222, 239
  HIV-related, 243–44, 245
dementia paralytica. *See* paresis
dementia praecox. *See* schizophrenia
depression, 6, 74, 106
  antidepressants for, 93, 135, 137,
    211–13
  gut microbes and, 97, 124, 129, 144
  hepatitis C and, 247
  malaria and, 202–3
  measurement of, 136–37
  See also bipolar disorder
Descartes, René, 17
despair, measurement of, 136–37
developing world
  drug supply in, 236–37, 247–50
  HIV/AIDS in, 242
  infection control in, 245–47
  infectious diseases in, 228–29, 237–45
  medical infrastructure in, 229–32
  schizophrenia in, 42, 70–71
  sleeping sickness in, 232–36
d'Herelle, Felix, 223
diabetes mellitus, 71, 148, 166
diet, 117, 151, 153–54
disease
  animal models of, 64–65, 68, 71, 113,
    136–38
  creation of, 140
  genetic models of, 6
  See also infectious diseases; mental
    disorders
disinfection procedures, 209, 210–11

dizygotic twins, 42–48
DNA, 45–46, 61, 62, 150
doctors vs. clergy, 17–18, 24–27, 28
Doctors Without Borders, 233–34, 236
Donizetti, Gaetano, 27
dopamine, 69–70, 135
doxycycline, 214
drugs. *See* medications
DSM (*Diagnostic and Statistical Manual of Mental Disorders*), 34, 35, 99, 104–6, 139, 152
dualism theory. *See* mind-body dualism

eating disorders, 92–93, 152
See also anorexia nervosa
Ebola virus, 199
Eckstein, Emma, 53, 54
efavirenz, 245
efference copy, 40
eflornithine, 235
Ehrlich, Paul, 28
Elliott, David, 217–18
Ellis, W. Gilmore, 163
Emami-Ahari, Dr., 118
emotions
animal models of, 136–37
gut microbes and, 142–43
encephalitis
anti-NMDA-receptor, 215, 217
measles and, 155–56
schizophrenia and, 12–13, 50
toxoplasmosis and, 66
von Economo's, 33, 56, 205
West Nile virus and, 109, 111
encephalitis lethargica, 33, 56, 205
encephalopathy, spongiform, 168, 238
endosymbiotic theory, 130–31
endotoxins, 145–46
enteric nervous system (ENS), 4, 129–30, 133, 134–35, 137
See also gut microbes
enterotypes, bacterial, 150–51
environment, 12, 34
genetics and, 43, 44
womb, 64–65, 71–72
epilepsy, 45, 241
Epstein-Barr virus, 51, 96
ergotism, 34, 206
Escherichia coli, 128

Esmark, Johannes Friedrich, 28
ethnocentrism, 164, 178
See also culture
evolution, 15, 126–27
human/microbial, 96, 198, 205–6, 216–17
microbial, 195, 197–98
Ewald, Paul, 5, 42–43, 74, 109, 195, 198–99, 200, 205, 207, 222
extroversion, 183

family dynamics, schizophrenia and, 38–39, 48–50, 115
Farmer, Paul, 225
fasting-induced adipose factor, 154
Fauci, Anthony, 254
Fazel, Seena, 41
fear
of infection, 177, 180–85
toxoplasma and, 187–89
fecal transplants, 157
Feck, Josef, 182
Fernández-Marina, Dr., 164
Ferraro, Armando, 142–43
fetal development
influenza infection in, 72–73
nervous system in, 133
schizophrenia origins in, 46–48, 64–65, 66, 68–69, 72, 208–9, 214–15
womb environment in, 71–72
fever, 222
Firmicutes, 150, 153–54
Fischer, Eugen, 182
Fischer, Martin H., 36–37
Fitzsimmons, Margery, 161
Flegr, Jaroslav, 68, 69–70
Fleming, John, 218
Fliess, William, 53
flu. *See* influenza
food poisoning, 33, 146
Fore people, 168–69, 238–39
Foucault, Michel, 17–18
Fournier, Jay, 211
Freud, Sigmund, 6–7, 18, 29–30, 51, 52, 53, 54
frigophobia, 164
Fromm-Reichmann, Frieda, 48, 51
fungi, 3, 16, 128

Gajdusek, Daniel Carleton, 238
GAS infections. *See* Group A
 streptococcal infections
Gates Foundation, 236, 237, 256
genetics, 6, 12, 74
 autism and, 141–42
 drug metabolism and, 245
 evolutionary success and, 127
 immunity and, 72, 108
 intelligence and, 116–17
 microbial, 132, 149–50
 mitochondrial, 130–31
 PANDAS and, 82, 86
 schizophrenia and, 15, 42–48, 72
genocide, 8
 conversion disorder and, 158–60
 culture-bound syndromes and,
  162–63
 infection model of, 169–73, 177–78,
  180–83
 South African apartheid and, 248
Genuis, Stephen J., 76
George III, King of England, 19–25
George IV, King of England, 22
German measles, 57, 70, 74, 237
germ theory, 4, 13, 210
 genetics and, 74
 paradigm shift to, 15, 31–35
 proof of causation based on, 107
 reaction to, 216
 second wave of, 5
Gershon, Michael, 6, 135, 141–42
Gilles de la Tourette, Georges, 89
Gisselquist, David, 246
Goethe, Johann Wolfgang von, 118
Goldberg, Rube, 26
gonorrhea, 205
Gordon, Jeffrey, 153–54
Gouge, Deborah, 231
Gould, Stephen Jay, 117
Griesinger, Wilhelm, 27
Group A streptococcal (GAS) infections
 anorexia and, 93, 94
 mental disorders related to, 6, 16–17,
  33, 84–86, 96
 obsessive-compulsive disorder and, 81,
  82, 85
 PANDAS and, 86–91, 95,
  101–2
 rheumatic fever and, 84, 85

Sydenham's chorea and, 83–84, 85,
 98, 101
 treatment of, 89–91
Grubber, William, 25
Guillain-Barré syndrome, 252, 254
gun violence, 171–72, 173
gut microbes, 3–4, 6, 125, 127–32
 autism and, 17, 144–47
 emotions, behavior, and, 136–38, 142–43
 enterotypes of, 150–51
 mental disorders linked to, 33, 124
 neonatal and infant, 132, 133–34
 obesity and, 151, 153–54
 transplants of, 157
 See also Helicobacter pylori; microbiome

HAART (highly active antiretroviral
 therapy), 214, 226–28, 243, 245
habit of thought, 8, 12, 112, 114–17
Hacking, Ian, 99, 100, 140–41
Hallett, Mark, 162
hand-washing, 209, 210–11
heart disease
 bacterial cause of, 6, 16, 96–97, 123
 fetal environment and, 71
 stress and, 102–3
Helicobacter pylori, 147–48
 obesity and, 131, 134, 148, 221
 protective role of, 131, 221
 ulcers and, 5–6, 16, 96, 117–22, 123, 147
Hemenway, David, 171–72, 173
hepatitis C virus, 5, 201, 247
herd immunity, 214, 222
herpes virus, 122
 schizophrenia and, 47, 64, 73–74, 208
 virulence of, 201, 206
HERV-W (human endogenous
 retrovirus W), 62–63, 64–65, 70, 82
Hess, Rudolf, 180
Hewison, Cathy, 233–34
Hill, Austin Bradford, 112
Himmler, Heinrich, 182
Hippocrates, 12
Hitler, Adolf, 27, 181–82
HIV/AIDS, 61, 63
 in developing world, 242–46
 drugs for, 214, 226–28, 243, 245
 fear of, 184–85
 mental effects of, 88
 virulence of, 199

HLAs (human leukocyte antigens), 72
Hofstede, Geert, 183
Holmes, Bayard Taylor, 54
Holmes, Ralph Loring, 54
Holocaust, 8, 169, 180–82
homelessness, 59
homicide, 178–79, 248
homosexuality, 99, 104–5
hopelessness, measurement of, 136–37
Hoppe-Seyler, Felix, 22
hospitals
    antiseptic techniques in, 208–11
    giving birth in, 245–46
    infection risk in, 206–8, 222
    mental, 17–18, 24, 27, 28
host, 96
    changing behavior of, 201–3
    density and mobility of, 199–201
Hotez, Peter, 256
human endogenous retrovirus W
        (HERV-W), 62–63, 64–65, 70, 82
human genome, 62, 132
human leukocyte antigens (HLAs), 72
Human Microbiome Project, 6, 149–51,
    221
human papillomavirus (HPV), 5, 16, 75,
    96, 122–23
Hutu people, 178, 182–83
Huxley, Aldous, 96, 135
Huxley, Thomas, 192
hygiene hypothesis, 216, 221
hypochondriasis, 102–3

iatrogenic infection, 23, 206–8, 222, 246
immune system, 4, 129–30, 133–34
    autism and, 141
    behavioral, 174–75, 176, 179
    evolution of, 216–17
    genetics and, 72, 108
    schizophrenia and, 64–65, 73, 214
    See also autoimmune diseases;
        PANDAS
immunization. See vaccines
India, drug industry in, 230–31,
    236–37
individualism, 183–84
infection control, 7–8, 207–11
    in developing world, 245–47, 249
    future of, 221–24
infection vs. contagion, 172–73

infectious diseases
    antibiotic-resistant, 196–97
    behavioral changes in, 36–37, 204–5
    carriers of, 108, 201
    collectivism vs. individualism and,
        183–84
    conquered, 32–33, 228, 249
    delayed onset of, 201
    detection of, 176–77
    in developing world, 228–29, 237–45
    fear of, 177, 180–85
    fighting one with another, 29–31
    genetics and, 72
    iatrogenic, 23, 206–8, 222, 246
    inflammation in, 65, 212–13
    linking microbes to, 4, 32
    mental disorders and, 5, 6–8, 13, 15–17,
        33–34, 43, 74–75, 87–88, 167–68
    opportunistic, 242, 244
    prevention of, 213–15, 222, 237
    proof of causation of, 107–9, 111–14
    psychosis in, 52–53
    revising response to, 221–24
    schizophrenia and, 44, 47, 50, 51–52
    seasonality of, 57–58
    transmission of, 199–201, 207, 245–47
    zoonotic, 13, 203–4
inflammation, 65, 74, 212–13, 218
influenza
    bipolar disorder and, 70, 72, 73
    in developing world, 247
    schizophrenia and, 16, 33, 47, 52,
        54–58, 64, 70, 72–74, 214–15
    vaccine for, 75, 206, 214, 222, 247
intelligence, genetics and, 116–17
interferon, 214
intestinal fortitude, 142
intestinal microbes. See gut microbes
irritable bowel syndrome, 135

Jabr, Ferris, 106
James I, King of England, 22
Jaworski, Walery, 118
Jenkins, Janis, 165–66
Jernigan, John, 210
Jessen W., 28
Jewish people, 180–82

Keane, Fergal, 183
Keim, Brandon, 173

Kempner, Joanna, 116, 117
Kendell, R. E., 12
Khmer women, 159–60, 162
Kilman, Joseph E., 142–43
Klitzman, Robert, 168, 238
Knaack, Stephanie, 100–101
knowledge, forbidden, 115, 116–17, 119, 123–24, 209
Koch, Robert, 4, 13, 32, 74, 107
Koch's postulates, 107–9, 111, 112, 113–14
kopi luwak (civet coffee), 186–87, 188
koro (genital-shrinking anxiety), 163
Kraepelin, Emil, 52
Krautwurst, Katie, 161
Kuchment, Anna, 223
Kufuor, John, 231
Kuhn, Thomas, 14–15, 36, 115
kuru (laughing sickness), 163, 167–69, 238–39
kynurenic acid, 149

labeling theory, 99
lactobacilli, 3, 128, 137, 148
Lactobacillus plantarum 299, 194–95
Laub, John, 172
leaky-gut syndrome, 141, 143–44
Lemoine, Bernard, 236
Lewis, Sinclair, 109
limbic encephalitides, 216
Lipkin, Ian, 65, 109–14, 242
lipopolysaccharides, 145
Loeffler, Friedrich, 4, 32, 107
Luhrmann, Tanya, 35, 48–49
Lund University, Sweden, 192–93
Lykoudis, John, 117, 118–19, 120, 121
lyssaviruses, 34

MacIntosh, Mary, 99
mad cow disease, 33, 123
Mahoney, John F., 31
malaria, 4
  cerebral, 202–3, 238
  in developing world, 228–29, 237–38
  genetic immunity to, 108
  schizophrenia and, 70
  treating syphilis with, 29–31, 100
  virulence of, 200, 201–3
Mallon, Mary (Typhoid Mary), 108, 201
Manceaux, Louis, 13

Manuelidis, Laura, 222, 232, 239
Marshall, Barry, 117–18, 120–21
Mary, Queen of Scots, 22
Massachusetts General Hospital, 38, 49
mass hysteria, 161–62
Masson, Jeffrey, 53
Maugham, W. Somerset, vii
Maupassant, Guy de, 27
Mayer, Emeran, 129
McGown, Richard, 248
McNeil, Thomas F., 71–72
measles, 33, 155–57
measles, mumps, rubella (MMR) vaccine, 154–55
medications, 33
  for developing world, 229–31, 235–37, 247–50
  mental effects of, 214, 226–28, 245
  murder using, 248
  for schizophrenia, 40, 42, 70, 75
melarsoprol, 234
Menninger, Karl, 12, 54–55
mental disorders
  advocacy for, 58–60
  autoimmune disease and, 216, 217
  childhood, 82, 84–87
  continuum concept of, 35
  culture-bound, 162–69
  dichotomy between physical and, 11–12, 17–19, 23–24, 28, 33, 34–35, 100–101
  DSM-5 definition of, 104
  Freud's conception of, 30
  gastrointestinal toxins and, 142–43, 144
  genetic cause of, 42–48
  genocide as, 169–73
  Group A streptococci and, 84–86, 96
  HIV and, 243–45
  infectious causes of, 5, 6–8, 13, 15–17, 33–34, 43, 74–75, 87–88, 167–68, 237–45
  influenza and, 55–56
  malaria and, 202–3
  measles and, 155–57
  multiple sclerosis as, 218–21
  obesity as, 152
  poverty and, 8, 224
  prevention of, 213–15
  stigma of, 98–101

mental disorders *(Cont.)*
  surgery for, 53–54
  taxonomy of, 25–26, 52
  trypanosomiasis and, 233–34
mental health care
  control of, 17–18, 24–27, 28
  misguided policies in, 58–59
Merrell Dow, 235
metabolic syndrome, 152
metabolism, 154, 245
miasmas, 4, 32
microbes, 3
  behavioral shaping by, 8, 136–38,
    142–43, 158, 174–80, 185–91, 201–3
  evolution of, 96, 195, 197–98
  fighting microbes with, 194–95
  hoarder, 153
  internal, 125, 127–32
  linking disease to, 4–6, 32
  mental disorders and, 6–8
  myopic tactics against, 206–8
  noninfectious diseases and, 5–6
  number of, 3, 125–26, 129, 132
  war with, 7–8, 126–27, 130, 198,
    216–17, 221–22
  See also bacteria; gut microbes;
    pathogens
microbiome, 3–4, 128–32
  mutation of, 134
  research on, 149–51
  See also gut microbes
milking sign, 84
Mills, Hannah, 24
mind
  Freud's structural theory of, 54
  species of, 11–12
mind-body dualism, 11–12
  clergy vs. physicians on, 23–24, 28
  DSM reinforcement of, 34–35
  mental illness stigma and, 100–101
  psychoactive drugs and, 33
  substance or Cartesian, 17–19
mitochondria, 130–31
Mix, Tom, 223
MMR (measles, mumps, rubella)
  vaccine, 154–55
molecular mimicry, 145–46
Mollica, Richard, 160
monozygotic twins, 42–48
moral failure, sickness as, 12, 98–101

moral treatment, 22, 24
morbillivirus, 204
Mortensen, Chad R., 174
mosquito, *Anopheles*, 4, 200, 201–2
  Aedes, 252, 255
mothers
  autism risk related to, 141
  hospital birthing for, 245–46
  medical conditions and behaviors in, 71
  schizophrenia risk related to, 48–52,
    64–65, 66, 68–69, 72–73, 207–8,
    214–15
Mukerji, Dr., 220–21
multiple personality disorder, 99
multiple sclerosis, 218–21
  B. fragilis and, 137–38, 141
  genetics and, 45
  immune response in, 64–65
  retroviruses and, 61–63
  seasonality of, 57–58
  whipworm infection and, 217, 218
murders, 178–79, 248
mutualism, 130, 131
Mycobacterium tuberculosis, 32, 204

Nabwire, Lutalo, 226, 227–28
National Alliance for the Mentally Ill, 58
National Institutes of Health, 76
Navarrete, Carlos, 175
Nazis, 71, 169, 180–82
neodissociation, 159
neologisms, 39
nervous system, 133
  efference copies produced by, 40
  enteric, 4, 129–30, 133, 134–35, 137
  See also brain
neural crest, 133
neurasthenia, 56, 72
neurocysticercosis, 241–42, 255
neuroimaging technologies, 61, 160
neurosyphilis, 10–11, 28
  See also syphilis
neurotransmitters
  enteric, 133, 135, 143
  schizophrenia and, 65, 69–70, 72
Nexavar, 236–37
Nicholson, Jeremy, 139, 144
Nicolle, Charles, 13
Nietzsche, Friedrich, 27
Noll, Richard, 53

NTDs, 253, 255, 256
Nutt, David, 230

obesity, 6, 151–54
    Firmicutes and, 151, 153–54
    Helicobacter pylori and, 131, 134, 148, 221
obsessive-compulsive disorder (OCD),
        5, 74
    anorexia and, 93
    Group A streptococci and, 6, 33, 84, 96
    PANDAS and, 86–87, 94, 95, 98, 101–2
    symptoms of, 80–83, 85–86, 90
    toxoplasmosis and, 70
Occam's razor, 96
opportunistic infections, 242, 244
Ornidyl, 235–36
ostracism, 179–80, 185

Packman, J., 240
PANDAS (pediatric autoimmune
        neuropsychiatric disorders
        associated with streptococcal
        infections), 79
    anorexia and, 91–94, 167
    biological cause of, 97–101
    controversy over, 101–4, 115–16
    disorders included in, 86–91
    DSM-5 and, 104–6
    Koch's postulates and, 108
    mass hysteria vs., 161–62
    mistaken identity of, 94–97
PANS (pediatric acute-onset
        neuropsychiatric syndrome), 104
Panum, Peter, 155
paradigm shift, 7, 15–17
    to germ theory, 15, 31–35
    resistance to, 35–36, 114, 124, 210
parasites, 16
    multicellular, 203, 204, 217–18, 240–43
    trypanosome, 232, 233
    See also malaria; *Toxoplasma gondii*
parasite-stress theory of sociality, 178
paresis
    influenza and, 55, 56
    syphilis and, 5, 10–11, 27–31, 33, 100,
        107, 112–13
Parkinson's syndrome, postencephalitic,
        56
Pasteur, Louis, 13, 32, 74, 209, 210, 216
pasteurization, 32

pathogenicity, 200
pathogens
    avoidance of, 174–75, 176–77
    depicting humans as, 180–82
    disease causation by, 107–8
    virulence of, 198–208, 222
    See also bacteria; microbes
patient vs. subject, 88
Patterson, Paul H., 47, 73, 141, 215
pediatric acute-onset neuropsychiatric
        syndrome (PANS), 104
    See also PANDAS
pellagra, 112–13
penicillin, 5, 31, 33, 231
pentamidine, 234
perfume, 185, 189–90
peripheral nervous system, 133
peristalsis, 134
Perron, Hervé, 61–62, 63, 64–65
Peters, Timothy J., 23
pharmaceutical industry, 229–31,
        235–37
phenotype, extended, 202–3
philopatric animals, 184
physical vs. mental disorders, 11–12,
        17–19, 23–24, 28,
        33, 34–35, 100–101
    See also infectious diseases
physicians vs. clergy, 17–18, 24–27, 28
pibloktoq (Arctic hysteria), 163
Pinker, Steven, 175
Pinsky, Drew (Dr. Drew), 161, 162
placenta, 46–47, 132
Planck, Max, 9
plasmodium. *See* malaria
plausibility, 112
pneumonia, ventilator-associated,
        192–93, 194–95
Pogo, 125, 128
poliomyelitis, 45, 108, 114, 249
poliovirus, 204, 206
Pollan, Michael, 157
poor and medically underserved
        population, 8, 224
porphyria, 22–23
Porsolt forced-swimming test, 136–37
Porter, Roy, 18
possible proof, 111, 113
Poussaint, Alvin F., 170, 172
pregnant women. *See* mothers

prejudice
  five-point scale of, 180
  protective, 174–75, 177, 183
  See also bias
prions, 16
  Creutzfeldt-Jakob disease and, 33, 108, 123, 168, 222
  kuru and, 238–39
prisons, racial bias in, 172
probable proof, 111, 113–14
probiotic supplements, 131–32, 148–49
Proctor, Lita, 128–29
proof of causation, 106
  Bradford Hill criteria for, 112–13
  categories for, 111, 113–14
  Koch's postulates for, 107–9
  resistance to, 117–23
Proteobacteria, 150
protozoa, 3, 128
Prusiner, Stanley, 123, 239
psychiatry
  community, 58–59
  culture vs., 171
  fashions in, 50, 99
  founders of, 25, 30, 52
  rejection of, 59–60
psychoanalysis, 30, 53, 54
psychosis, 7, 41
  cultural bias in labeling, 105
  HIV-related, 243–45
  infectious diseases with, 52–53
  influenza and, 54, 55
  See also schizophrenia
puerperal infection, 32, 209

Quakers, 24–25
quinolones, 118
quorum sensing, 193–94

rabies, 34, 113, 202, 203
racial violence, 169–70, 173
  See also genocide
racism, 172, 176, 180, 248
Raes, Jeroen, 125, 128, 131–32, 150–51
Raleigh, Sir Walter, 38
religious orders vs. doctors, 17–18, 24–27, 28
retroviruses, 61–64
rheumatic fever, 83, 84, 85, 86, 101
Richardson, Sir Benjamin Ward, 56

Rigoni-Stern, Domenico Antonio, 122
Rin, Hsien, 164
RNA, 61
roundworms, 203, 204, 242
rubella, 57, 70, 74, 237, 253
Rush, Benjamin, 25–27
Rwandan genocide, 169, 178, 182–83

Sacks, Oliver, 244
Salmonella typhimurium, 201, 205
Salvarsan, 28
Sapolsky, Robert, 168–69, 175, 187–88
scent, microbial role in, 185–91
Schaller, Mark, 174
schizoaffective disorder, 44
schizophrenia, 5, 7, 38–42
  autism and, 139
  autoantibodies in, 216
  brain in, 51, 65, 70, 72, 73
  collectivist worldview and, 184
  cultural variations of, 165–66
  fetal origins of, 64–65, 71–72
  genetics and, 15, 42–48, 72, 115
  historical background on, 52–55
  infectious causes of, 16, 33, 47, 50, 51–52, 64, 70–71, 74, 207–8
  influenza and, 55–57, 72–74, 214–15
  medications for, 40, 42, 70, 75
  psychosocial causes of, 38–39, 48–50, 115
  retroviruses and, 61–64
  rubella and, 237
  seasonality of, 57–58, 61
  toxoplasmosis and, 13–14, 66–71
  viral encephalitis and, 12–13
Schumann, Robert, 27
seasonality
  of schizophrenia, 57–58, 61
  of Sydenham's chorea, 84
selective serotonin reuptake inhibitors (SSRIs), 135, 211–13
Semmelweis, Ignaz, 209–10
Semmelweis reflex, 210
serotonin, 135, 213
sexual attraction, 187–89
sexually transmitted diseases (STDs), 31, 100, 205
  See also syphilis
sexual orientation disturbance, 105
Shrira, Ilan, 175, 178–79

sickle-cell trait, 108
sickness behavior, 36–37, 204–5
Simpson, William, 155
Sims, James Marion, 122
Singer, Harvey, 103, 104
Sjoerdsma, Albert, 234–35
Skelly, David, 177
sleeping sickness, 231, 232–36, 247
Slutkin, Gary, 173
smallpox virus, 32–33, 199
Soon, Chun Siong, 35
South Sudan, Republic of, 169
Spering, Miriam, 40
SSPE (subacute sclerosing
    panencephalitis), 155–56
SSRIs (selective serotonin reuptake
    inhibitors), 135, 211–13
Stalin, Josef, 223
Stanley Medical Research Institute, 51, 60
St. Anthony's fire, 4, 34
staphylococci, 3, 128, 137, 148–49
Starling, Ernest H., 134
statistical significance, 212
STDs (sexually transmitted diseases),
    31, 100, 205
    See also syphilis
Stewart, William, 196
stigma, 31, 98–101
stomach cancer, 118, 147
Strachan, David P., 216
streptococcal infections. *See* Group A
    streptococcal infections
streptomycin, 231
stress, 42, 74
    heart disease and, 102–3
    lactobacilli and, 148
    ulcers and, 117
Structure of Scientific Revolutions,
    The (Kuhn), 14–15, 115
St. Vitus's Dance, 83, 85
subacute sclerosing panencephalitis
    (SSPE), 155–56
subject vs. patient, 88
substance dualism, 17–19
suramin, 234
surgery, 53–54
Swango, Michael, 248
Swedo, Susan, 6, 76–79, 83–91, 94–96,
    98, 101, 103, 104, 115–16, 161–62
Sydenham, Thomas, 83

Sydenham's chorea, 83–85, 87
    genetic susceptibility to, 86
    Group A streptococci and, 98, 101
    PANDAS and, 94, 95–96
symbiosis, 130, 131
syphilis, 9–11
    paresis in, 5, 28–31, 100, 107, 112–13
    virulence of, 205
systemic lupus erythematosus, 221
Szasz, Thomas, 59–60

Taenia solium (pork tapeworm), 241–42
Tagamet, 117, 118, 119, 121
"talking cure," 30, 53, 54
tastes, microbial role in, 8, 185–91
Taylor, Elizabeth, 223
Tay-Sachs disease, 108
T cells, 65, 217–18
temporality, 113
testosterone, 187, 189
tetracycline, 103
Third Reich, 180–82
Third World. *See* developing world
Thomas, Lewis, 200
Thornhill, Randy, 177–78, 183–84
tics, 84, 86, 88–89, 96
    See also Tourette's syndrome
Torrey, Edwin Fuller, 6–7, 13, 14, 38–39,
    44, 47, 49–52, 56–64, 66, 67, 68, 69,
    70–71, 72, 73–74
Torrey, Rhoda, 38–39, 49–50
Tourette's syndrome, 5, 89–90
    genetics and, 82
    Group A streptococci and, 6, 16–17, 33,
    86, 96
    PANDAS and, 86–87, 94, 95–96, 98,
    101–2
Toxocara canis, 203, 204, 242
Toxoplasma gondii, 33
    animals infected by, 204
    defensive enzyme of, 198
    host manipulation by, 202, 203
    prevention of, 222
    schizophrenia and, 13–14, 47, 51–52,
    64, 66–71, 74, 208
    tastes, scent, and, 185–91
tranquilizing chair, 26
trauma
    mental disorders and, 12, 16, 42, 74, 115
    obesity and, 152

Treponema pallidum, 28, 113, 199
  See also syphilis
trichinosis, 240–41
triclosan, 211
Trifiletti, Rosario, 161–62
trypanosomiasis, 231, 232–36, 247
tuberculosis, 32, 100, 108, 204
Tuke, William, 24
Turk, Jim, 218
Tutsi people, 178, 182–83
twin studies, 42–48, 72
twin-to-twin transfusion syndrome, 46–47
Tynan, Ross, 212–13
typhoid, 108, 201
Typhoid Mary (Mary Mallon), 108, 201

ulcerative colitis, 217, 218
ulcers, *Helicobacter pylori* and, 5–6, 16,
  96, 117–22, 123, 147
Unger, Thomas, 100–101
United Nations (UN), 231, 245

vaccines
  autism and, 140, 144
  for developing world, 247–49
  HPV, 75, 122
  influenza, 75, 206, 214, 222, 247
  measles, 154–55, 157
  polio, 108, 114
  rubella, 70
  toxoplasmosis, 71
vagus nerve, 129, 133, 134, 135, 137
Van Boemel, Gretchen, 158–59
vancomycin, 146
Vaniqa, 236
Van Nieuwenhove, Simon, 235
venereal disease, 31, 100, 205
  See also syphilis
ventilator-associated pneumonia (VAP),
  192–93, 194–95
Vibrio cholerae, 205
violence, 8
  infection model of, 169–73, 177–79
  schizophrenia and, 40–41
  See also genocide
virulence, 198–206
  hospitals as incubators of, 206–8
  manipulation of, 222
viruses, 3, 16, 111
  antibiotics and, 197

bacteriophage, 197, 223–24
  intestinal, 128
  retroviruses, 61–64
  See also specific species
  vitamin production, 131
Vogel, Dr., 80–81
von Economo's encephalitis, 33, 56, 205
Vyas, Ajai, 187

Wagner-Jauregg, Julius, 28–29, 30, 31
Wain, Louis, 14
Warren, Robin, 117–18, 120–21
Wassermann tests, 28
water, pathogens in, 206
Weinstock, Joel V., 217
West Nile virus, 109, 111
whipworms, 217–18
whooping cough, 156
Wilce, John, 142
William of Occam, 96
Williams, Daniel Hale, 122
Williams, George C., 126, 127
Williams, Kipling D., 179
Willis, Rev. Francis, 20–22, 23, 24
Windigo psychosis, 164–65
wine, 185, 190–91
World Health Organization (WHO), 42,
  231, 242, 243, 246, 252
World Trade Organization (WTO), 231
worldview, 15, 127, 183–84
worms, intestinal, 203, 204, 217–18,
  240–43

Xavier, Ramnik Joseph, 131–32, 148, 151
xenophobia, 8, 175, 176, 177–79, 184

Yadegaran, Jessica, 190
Yersinia pestis, 205
Yolken, Robert, 7, 14, 51–52, 56–57,
  61–64, 67–73, 237, 240
York Retreat, 24
Young, Ry, 223

Zadro, Lisa, 179
Zika virus, 251–57
Zinsser, Han, 126
Zobellia galactanivorans, 151
zoonotic infections, 13, 203–4
Županc, Tatjana Avšič, 252
zur Hausen, Harald, 122

About the Author

Harriet A. Washington, the Shearing Fellow at the University of Nevada's Black Mountain Institute, has been a research fellow in medical ethics at Harvard Medical School and a senior research scholar at the National Center for Bioethics at Tuskegee University, as well as a visiting scholar at DePaul University College of Law. She has held a visiting fellowship at the Harvard School of Public Health and a John S. Knight Fellowship at Stanford University. She wrote *Deadly Monopolies* and *Medical Apartheid,* which won the National Book Critics Circle Award, the PEN Oakland Award, the Gustavus Myers Award, and the Black Caucus of the American Library Association Nonfiction Award.